Lyme Disease

Lyme
Disease

■ ■ ■

Daniel W. Rahn, MD, FACP, FACR
Professor of Medicine
Chief, Section of General Internal Medicine
Vice Dean for Clinical Affairs
Medical College of Georgia
Augusta, GA

Janine Evans, MD
Assistant Professor of Medicine
Yale University School of Medicine
New Haven, CT

A|C|P

American College of Physicians
Philadelphia, Pennsylvania

Acquisitions Editor: Mary K. Ruff
Manager, Book Publishing: David Myers
Administrator, Book Publishing: Diane M. McCabe
Production Supervisor: Allan S. Kleinberg
Production Editor: Victoria Hoenigke
Development Editor: Michael G. Bokulich
Interior Design: Kate Nichols
Cover Design: Elizabeth Swartz

Printed in the United States of America.
Composition by Fulcrum Data Services, Inc.
Printing/binding by Versa Press.

American College of Physicians
Independence Mall West
Sixth Street at Race
Philadelphia, PA 19106-1572

Library of Congress Cataloging-in-Publication Data

Lyme disease / [edited by] Daniel Rahn, Janine Evans.
   p. cm. -- (Key diseases series ; 1) Includes bibliographical
   references.
   ISBN 0-943126-58-4 (alk. paper)
   1. Lyme disease. I. Rahn, Daniel, 1950- . II. Evans, Janine, 1955- . III. Series.
   [DNLM: 1. Lyme Disease. WC 406 L9856 1998]
RC155.5.L942 1998
616.9'2--dc21
DNLM/DLC
for Library of Congress   97-3304
                                                   CIP

99 00 01 02 03 / 9 8 7 6 5 4 3

Contributors

David T. Dennis, MD, MPH
Chief, Bacterial Zoonoses Branch
Division of Vector–Borne Infectious
  Diseases
National Center for Infectious
  Diseases
Centers for Disease Control
Fort Collins, CO

Janine Evans, MD
Assistant Professor of Medicine
Yale University School of Medicine
New Haven, CT

Erol Fikrig, MD
Associate Professor of Medicine
Yale University School of Medicine
New Haven, CT

Eric L. Logigian, MD
Associate Professor of Neurology
Harvard Medical School
Director of Clinical
  Neurophysiology at Brigham and
  Women's Hospital
Boston, MA

Robert B. Nadelman, MD
Associate Professor of Medicine
Division of Infectious Diseases
Westchester County Medical Center/
  New York Medical College
Valhalla, NY

**Daniel W. Rahn, MD, FACP,
  FACR**
Professor of Medicine
Chief, Section of General Internal
  Medicine
Vice Dean for Clinical Affairs
Medical College of Georgia
Augusta, GA

Robert T. Schoen, MD
Clinical Professor of Medicine
Yale University School of Medicine
New Haven, CT

Eugene D. Shapiro, MD
Professor of Pediatrics and of
  Epidemiology and Public Health
Yale University School of Medicine
  and the Children's Clinical
  Research Center
New Haven, CT

Leonard H. Sigal, MD, FACP, FACR
Chief, Division of Rheumatology
University of Medicine and
  Dentistry of New Jersey
Robert Wood Johnson
  Medical School
New Brunswick, NJ

Anthony D. So, MD, MPA
Senior Advisor to the Administrator
Agency for Health Care, Policy,
  and Research
U.S. Department of Health and
  Human Services
Washington, DC

Allen C. Steere, MD
Professor of Medicine
Tufts University School of Medicine
New England Medical Center
Boston, MA

Gary P. Wormser, MD
Chief, Division of Infectious
  Diseases
Professor of Medicine and
  Pharmacology
New York Medical College
Valhalla, NY

Contents

Introduction

Daniel W. Rahn, MD

Janine Evans, MD

L yme disease was first recognized as a distinct disease in 1975, when a group of concerned parents alerted the Connecticut State Health Department about an epidemic of inflammatory arthritis in their children in the region around Lyme, Connecticut (1). Some of the affected children had been diagnosed to have juvenile rheumatoid arthritis (JRA), a distinctly rare disorder not known to occur in epidemic fashion. A large number of children in this sparsely populated, rural region had been diagnosed to have JRA, resulting in an apparent attack rate that was unlike anything reported in the medical literature. The problem was referred to physicians in the rheumatology section at Yale University School of Medicine, who undertook a retrospective, community-based survey to determine whether the clinical and epidemiologic features of this new illness could be characterized.

The initial landmark retrospective study, conducted between December 1975 and April 1976, uncovered 51 persons (39 children and 12 adults) from the contiguous southern Connecticut communities of Old Lyme, Lyme, and East Haddam, who had arthritis typified by brief, recurrent episodes of swelling of one to a few large joints, most often the knee. Seventeen of the 39 affected children lived on one of four particular rural roads. The first case had occurred in 1972 in Lyme, for which the new syndrome, Lyme arthritis, was named.

Most of the cases began in summer months. This seasonality, combined with the clustering of the cases and epidemiologic analysis, suggested an arthropod vector. In addition, 25% of affected persons described an expanding annular skin lesion before the onset of the arthritis. This skin lesion was consistent with the entity erythema chronicum migrans, previously associated with an arthropod bite but not arthritis (2). On the basis of these suggestive, retrospectively collected data, further epidemiologic and prospective clinical studies were planned. The goals were to complete the clinical description and identify an infectious agent that could conceivably be causing this new illness.

A surveillance system was organized among physicians in practice in the endemic region. A prospective study in the spring and summer of 1976 led to the identification of 32 additional cases with the skin lesion ($n = 5$), arthritis ($n = 8$), or both ($n = 19$) (3). Of the 12 patients seen and examined at the time that they had active skin lesions, 6 had multiple skin lesions. Three patients recalled having been bitten by a tick at the site of the initial skin lesion 4, 14, and 20 days before onset of their skin lesion, respectively. The skin lesion was proved conclusively to be erythema chronicum migrans, which had been described more than a half a century earlier in Sweden but had not previously been described in the United States and was not known to be associated with arthritis. When the two occurred in the same person, the skin lesion always preceded the arthritis (by a median of 4 weeks). In addition, multiple flu-like symptoms occurred in association with the skin lesion(s), including headache, stiff neck, arthralgia, myalgia, fatigue, fever, lymphadenopathy, nausea, and even vomiting.

The arthritis was characterized by brief (average, 8 days) recurrent attacks of inflammation and swelling of one to a few joints, most often the knee. The onset of the arthritis varied in relation to skin lesions, occurring while lesions were still present to as late as 5 months after. Other clinical features emerged in this second study. Four patients had neurologic abnormalities, including 2 with Bell palsy, one of whom had a radiculopathy, and 2 with lymphocytic meningitis. Of 23 other patients with skin lesions on whom complete information was available, 12 had fever, headache, and stiff neck suggestive of aseptic meningitis. Similar findings were noted in 4 of 8 patients with arthritis that was not preceded by skin lesions. Two patients developed fluctuating, self-limited atrioventricular heart block. Detailed viral and bacterial cultures were all negative. Many patients had cryoglobulins during periods of active inflammation (4).

What emerged was a picture of a multisystem disease that evolved over weeks to months, probably associated with an infectious agent transmitted through a tick bite and associated with prominent immunologic phenomena. In recognition of the multisystem nature of the disease, the name was changed to Lyme disease.

The next few years were devoted to studies focused on isolating an infectious agent, further characterizing the epidemiology and vector ecology, and empirical treatment trials. Epidemiologic studies discovered a newly unidentified ixodid tick in the endemic region (5,6); this tick (originally named *Ixodes dammini* but subsequently shown to be a subspecies of *Ixodes scapularis*) (7) was then shown conclusively to be the vector of Lyme disease.

Preliminary information had suggested that erythema chronicum migrans might be responsive to penicillin and tetracycline or both (8). From 1980 to 1982, patients were enrolled in an open-label, randomized trial comparing penicillin, erythromycin, and tetracycline for the treatment of erythema chronicum migrans. All three treatments shortened the duration of this disorder compared with untreated historical controls and, more significantly, reduced progression to later stages of disease by preventing subsequent arthritis, carditis, and neurologic abnormalities (9). Erythromycin was less effective than the other agents, and in a significant minority of these patients arthralgias and fatigue developed during the course of the illness. These symptoms did not appear to respond to the short-course, low-dose antibiotics used in the trial but in most cases gradually resolved after several months.

Parenteral penicillin in a regimen known to be effective for secondary syphilis (bicillin, 2.4 MU intramuscularly weekly for 3 weeks) was tried empirically for the treatment of patients with arthritis, again with intermediate results. Seven of 20 patients who were treated had cessation of their episodes of arthritis. Intravenous penicillin for 10 days was slightly more effective (10). These results suggested strongly that Lyme disease was caused by an infectious agent that was susceptible to a variety of antibiotics. The disease course, which evolved in stages from localized to disseminated and then to chronically persistent inflammation over weeks to months, and the range of antibiotics to which the organism appeared to be responsive suggested a spirochete. In 1982 a previously unrecognized spirochete was cultured from *I. scapularis* ticks on Shelter Island, New York, an area known to be endemic for Lyme disease. Nine patients with Lyme disease were shown by immunofluorescence assay to have high antibody titers against this organism (11). Shortly thereafter, the same organism was isolated from blood, skin, and cerebrospinal fluid of patients with Lyme disease, and the full antibody response was characterized by enzyme-linked immunosorbent assay and then Western blot (12,13). The organism was most similar to previously identified borreliae in that it was tick transmitted and could be grown in artificial media; none of the other spirochetes pathogenic for humans could be grown in culture. It was named *Borrelia burgdorferi* after Dr. Willy Burgdorfer, who isolated and characterized the organism.

Since the early 1980s, many of the gaps in knowledge about Lyme disease have been filled in, resulting in a much more complete picture of the illness. Information has emerged in a fashion that has mirrored medical progress in general. The focus of research efforts has progressed from population-based, observational studies to detailed studies of the mechanisms underlying the specific interaction between the causative organism and the human host. Although the initial studies of Lyme disease consisted primarily of clinical descriptions and epidemiologic observations, they laid the foundation for current research into the molecular genetics of the causative organism. It is expected that ongoing research efforts will provide answers to nagging questions about disease persistence and clinical variability.

A better scientific understanding of Lyme disease will only go part way, however, in addressing the issues clinicians must face in evaluating and treating persons with Lyme disease or Lyme disease–like complaints. Many day-to-day dilemmas relate to physician and patient expectations and concerns about the risks and benefits of treating versus not treating when faced with clinical uncertainty. This monograph is intended to provide practicing physicians with a useful guide to bridge the gap between medical knowledge and clinical decision making. It includes chapters focusing on common clinical manifestations of Lyme disease and current best practice, as well as a separate section of clinical vignettes representing the range of problems often confronted in clinical practice. It is our hope that clinicians will find this approach useful in their daily practice of medicine.

REFERENCES

1. **Steere AC, Malawista SE, Syndman DR, et al.** Lyme arthritis: an epidemic of oligoarticular arthritis in children and adults in three Connecticut communities. Arthritis Rheum. 1977;20:7-17.

2. **Afzelius A.** Erythema chronicum migrans. Acta Derm Venereol suppl (Stockh). 1921;2:120.

3. **Steere AC, Malawista SE, Hardin JA, et al.** Erythema chronicum migrans and Lyme arthritis. Ann Intern Med. 1977;86:695-8.

4. **Steere AC, Hardin JA, Ruddy S, et al.** Lyme arthritis: correlation of serum and cryoglobulin IgM with activity, and serum IgG with remission. Arthritis Rheum. 1979;22:471-83.

5. **Steere AC, Broderick TF, Malawista SE.** Erythema chronicum migrans and Lyme arthritis: epidemiologic evidence of a tick vector. Am J Epidemiol. 1979;108:312-21.

6. **Steere AC, Malawista SE.** Cases of Lyme disease in the United States: locations correlated with distribution of *Ixodes dammini.* Ann Intern Med. 1979;91:730-3.

7. **Oliver JH, Owsley MR, Hutcheson HJ, et al.** Conspecificity of the ticks *Ixodes scapularis* and *I. dammini* (Acari: Ixodidae). J Med Entomol. 1993;30:54-63.

8. **Steere AC, Malawista SE, Newman JII, et al.** Antibiotic therapy in Lyme disease. Ann Intern Med. 1980;93:1-8.

9. **Steere AC, Hutchinson GJ, Rahn DW, et al.** Treatment of the early manifestations of Lyme disease. Ann Intern Med. 1983;99:22-6.

10. **Steere AC, Greene J, Schoen RT, et al.** Successful parenteral penicillin therapy of established Lyme arthritis. N Engl J Med. 1985;312:869-74.

11. **Steere AC, Grodzicki RL, Kornblatt AN, et al.** The spirochetal etiology of Lyme disease. N Engl J Med. 1983;308:76-82.
12. **Craft JE, Grodzicki RL, Steere AC.** Antibody response in Lyme disease: evaluation of diagnostic tests. J Infect Dis. 1984;78:934-9.
13. **Craft JE, Fischer DK, Shimamoto GT, Steere AC.** Antigens of *Borrelia burgdorferi* recognized during Lyme disease. J Clin Invest. 1986;78:934-9.

1

■ ■ ■

Epidemiology, Ecology, and Prevention of Lyme Disease

David T. Dennis, MD, MPH

Lyme disease is a rapidly emerging, vector-borne infectious disease in the United States and in wide areas of Europe and Asia. More than 95,000 cases have been reported to health authorities in the United States since 1982, when a systematic national surveillance was initiated. Lyme disease now accounts for more than 95% of all reported vector-borne illness in the United States.

The overall incidence of reported cases in the United States is approximately 5 per 100,000 persons, but there is considerable under-reporting. The disease occurs in distinct and geographically limited foci. The incidence in a few of the most highly endemic communities may be as high as 1% to 3% per year. Persons of all ages and both sexes are equally susceptible, although the highest attack rates are in children up to 14 years old and in persons 30 years of age and older. Although cases of Lyme disease have been reported from 48 states, a high incidence of infection is found in only about 80 counties in eight states located along the northeastern and mid-Atlantic seaboard, in Wisconsin and Minnesota, and in a few counties in northern California.

Vaccines to protect against the agent of Lyme disease, *Borrelia burgdorferi*, are in the final stages of evaluation, and new strategies of tick control are being developed. However, personal protection to avoid tick bites, early detection and removal of attached ticks, early diagnosis and treatment of disease, and environmental management of residential properties remain the cornerstones of prevention.

Etiologic Agent

The Lyme Disease Spirochete

European physicians described a form of erythema migrans (EM) in the early part of the century, associated this rash with tick bites, and postulated that it was caused by a tick-borne nonpyogenic bacterium responsive to penicillin (1). Scrimenti (2), aware of these findings, diagnosed EM in a patient in Wisconsin in 1969 and successfully treated the illness with penicillin. During the mid-1970s, studies of Lyme arthritis in Connecticut by Steere and colleagues (3,4) also linked the presence of EM to antecedent tick bites and determined that early treatment with penicillin not only shortened the duration of EM but reduced the risk of subsequent arthritis (5).

In 1982, Burgdorfer (6) identified spirochetes in the midgut of the adult deer tick, *Ixodes dammini* (renamed as *Ixodes scapularis*), and Barbour (7) cultured the spirochete in a modified Kelly's medium (BSK). Spirochetes were then cultured from blood samples of patients with EM, from tissue samples taken from the rash lesion itself, and from cerebrospinal fluid samples of a patient with meningoencephalitis and history of previous EM (8,9). The spirochete isolated from ticks and humans was described by Johnson and colleagues in 1984 (10) as *Borrelia burgdorferi*.

Borrelia, including *B. burgdorferi*, are flexible helical cells composed of a protoplasmic cylinder surrounded by a cell membrane, 7 to 11 periplasmic flagella, and an outer membrane that is loosely associated with the underlying structures (Fig. 1.1) (11). The outer membrane of *B. burgdorferi* and other *Borrelia* spp. is unique in that genes encoding its proteins are lo-

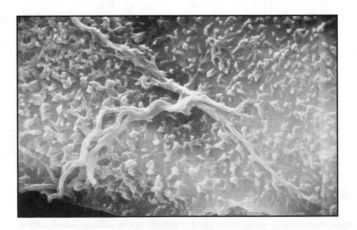

Figure 1.1   Electron micrograph of Lyme disease spirochetes, *Borrelia burgdorferi*, showing loose coils.

cated on linear plasmids; these extrachromosomal genes determine the antigenic identity of these organisms and are responsible for adaptive antigenic variation.

B. burgdorferi is made up of at least 30 different immunogenic proteins (12), including three major outer-surface proteins, OspA (30 kd), OspB (34 kd), and OspC (23 kd). The 41-kd antigen, similar to that of other spirochetes, is located on the flagellum. Other prominent antigens include the 18, 28, 35, 37, 39, 45, 58, 66, and 93-kd antigens.

Several genetic differences have been described within and between isolates of B. burgdorferi genospecies from Europe and the United States (13,14). The strain infecting humans in the United States is designated B. burgdorferi sensu stricto. Although this strain also infects humans in Europe, the two dominant genospecies in Europe are Borrelia garinii and Borrelia afzelii (15).

Evidence is accumulating that the different genospecies are associated with somewhat different disease expressions (16,17). Arthritis appears to occur more commonly after infection with B. burgdorferi sensu stricto; neurologic manifestations are believed to be more common after infection with B. garinii; and various cutaneous manifestations occur more commonly in association with B. afzelii infection.

Transmission of Infection to Humans

Lyme disease spirochetes are transmitted through the saliva of feeding ticks and possibly by regurgitation of tick midgut contents into the bite site. There is no evidence that B. burgdorferi is passed directly from one person to another. Infection is not known to be transmitted by sexual contact or through breast milk.

Transplacental infection of the fetus has been suggested by the finding of rare silver-stained spirochetal structures in fetal tissues (18), but this finding has not been adequately confirmed by cultural isolation and bacterial characterization. Although B. burgdorferi can be cultured from the blood in a small percentage of patients with early acute infection and is able to survive in stored blood for prolonged periods, transfusion-acquired infection has not been documented (19).

Human–Spirochete Interaction

Lyme disease is a multiphase, multisystem, tick-borne zoonosis that is categorized into early localized, early disseminated, and late disseminated stages (20). The portal of entry of B. burgdorferi is the dermis, at the site of infective tick attachment. After inoculation, infection spreads through cutaneous, lymphatic, and hematogenous extension.

An incubation period of 3 to 30 days (typically 7 to 14 days) occurs between the time of infection and onset of EM. The expanding, annular, erythematous rash, which occurs in 70% or more of cases, is usually accompanied by mild constitutional symptoms and occasionally by regional lymphadenitis. Not all patients remember having a rash or other early symptoms, and weeks or months may elapse before later-stage manifestations are recognized. The latent period may also vary from days to weeks.

B. burgdorferi can be cultured from 80% or more of biopsy specimens taken from early EM lesions (21). IgM antibodies to *B. burgdorferi* can be detected within 1 to 2 weeks after EM onset in 40% or more of patients and usually peak between the third and sixth weeks of illness. IgG responses may arise early or be delayed for weeks (22,23).

Patients with early disseminated disease, such as cranial neuritis or multiple EM, and those with active later-stage disease, such as arthritis, radiculoneuritis, meningoencephalitis, or acrodermatitis chronicum atrophicans, almost always have strong seroreactivity to *B. burgdorferi* antigens (23,24). In patients with early localized disease, antibiotic treatment may blunt or abrogate the immune response, and only about 60% of persons who receive early treatment develop serologic confirmation of infection. Seronegative late-stage Lyme disease does occur, but it is believed to be infrequent (25,26). Infection does not confer lasting protective immunity, and more than one occurrence of primary EM is not uncommon among persons at high environmental risk (27,28).

Untreated and inadequately treated infection may result in microbial persistence, and *B. burgdorferi* has been isolated from skin lesions, myocardium, synovial fluid, and cerebrospinal fluid samples months and years after the onset of symptoms (29–32). Subclinical infection is probably common (33,34). Genetic differences in susceptibility to infection have not been described, but chronic, refractory Lyme arthritis is associated with the major histocompatibility antigen, HLA-DR4 (35).

Although morbidity may (infrequently) be severe, chronic, and disabling, especially if the disease is not treated in its early stages, Lyme disease is rarely, if ever, fatal. No deaths caused by Lyme disease, fetal or otherwise, confirmed by cultural isolation of *B. burgdorferi* have been reported. Maternal Lyme disease is not a proven cause of intrauterine death or congenital malformations, although this association has been suggested (36). Epidemiologic studies do not show a correlation between Lyme disease endemicity and rates of adverse events of pregnancy (37).

Concurrent Lyme disease and babesiosis have been associated with a severity and duration of illness greater than that expected for either disease alone (38), and a case of fatal pancarditis in which spirochetal structures were seen in the myocardium was reported in a patient who had both Lyme disease and babesiosis (39). The importance of differentiating illness caused by *Borrelia*, *Babesia*, *Ehrlichia*, and other, as yet unidentified, agents transmitted by the same tick vectors has recently been highlighted (40).

Ecology of the Lyme Disease Spirochete

Natural Cycle of Infection

Lyme borreliosis is a zoonotic infection. Humans are incidental hosts of *B. burgdorferi* and do not contribute to its maintenance in nature. The basic elements in the life cycle of *B. burgdorferi* in North America are as follows (41,42) (Fig. 1.2):

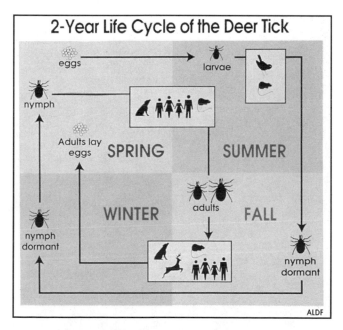

Figure 1.2   Life cycle of Lyme disease ticks in the eastern United States. The white-footed mouse is the principal host for black-legged (deer) tick larvae, which feed in late summer, and for the nymphs, which feed in late spring and early summer. Most Lyme disease in humans is acquired by the bites of the small-sized nymphal ticks. Adult black-legged ticks are much less likely than nymphs to transmit Lyme disease. (Courtesy of American Lyme Disease Foundation, Somers, NY.)

- Small rodents, especially the white-footed mouse *(Peromyscus leucopus)* and the chipmunk in the northeastern and northcentral states and the dusky wood rat (pack rat) and kangaroo rat in the Pacific coastal regions, serve as the principal reservoirs of *B. burgdorferi* infection for vector ticks.

- Three stages of vector ticks (larva, nymph, and adult) (Fig. 1.3/Plate 1) are involved in a 2-year life cycle, and each stage normally takes a single blood meal.

- Transstadial transmission of *B. burgdorferi* from larvae to nymphs and from nymphs to adults helps maintain the infective cycle, while transmission from an infected adult female to her eggs (transovarial transmission) rarely occurs.

- The efficiency of the transmission cycle is enhanced in eastern regions by sequential tick-feeding patterns—i.e., nymphs, feeding in the spring, infect rodents that in turn serve as sources of infection for larvae, which hatch and feed in the summer months.

- Deer, especially the white-tailed deer, *Odocoileus virginianus*, and other large- and medium-sized animals, serve as a mating ground for adult ticks and provide adult female ticks the blood

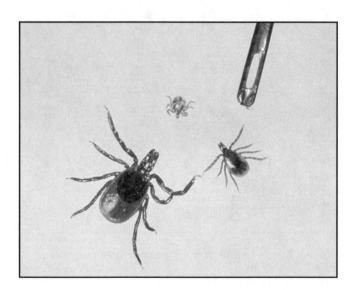

Figure 1.3 The three life forms (larva, nymph, adult) of unfed *Ixodes scapularis*, the black-legged (deer) tick. Their sizes are shown relative to the eye of a sewing needle. Nymphs, which feed during late spring and early summer, are responsible for most cases of Lyme disease. (Courtesy of Russell C. Johnson, PhD, University of Minnesota.) (For color reproduction, see Plate 1 at back of book.)

meal required for egg production. Deer are incompetent reservoirs of *B. burgdorferi* (43,44).

In the eastern and northcentral United States, humans are most often infected by the bite of nymphal-stage ticks. Some of the reasons for this are as follows:

1. Infected nymphs are present in large numbers in endemic areas in the late spring and summer months, when persons are active out-of-doors and lightly clothed.
2. Nymphs are minute and easily overlooked, especially when they attach in hirsute or other hard-to-observe areas of the body.
3. Unlike nymphs, adult ticks seek blood meals mostly in the late fall, winter, and early spring, when human outdoor activities are limited and additional clothing prevents access to skin.
4. Adult ticks are larger, more easily spotted, and more likely to be removed before transmission occurs than nymphs.

Global Distribution of Lyme Disease and Its Tick Vectors

Persons with Lyme disease are found in the range of *I. ricinus* complex ticks throughout temperate regions in North America, Europe, and Asia (Fig. 1.4) (41,45). Enzootic *B. burgdorferi* areas include portions of the United States and Canada, the British Isles, Scandinavia, western and central Europe, Balkan states, and states of the former Soviet Union, from the Baltics east through the northern forested areas of Russia to the Pacific coast and Japan (46–48).

In China, the disease is most endemic in forested northeastern regions and occurs with lower endemicity in widely scattered foci elsewhere in the country (49). Cases also occur sporadically in Japan (42,50). In the highly endemic areas of Europe and Asia, the incidence and epidemiologic patterns of Lyme disease are similar to those reported in North America (51).

I. scapularis is the principal vector in the eastern United States, and *I. pacificus*, the western black-legged tick, transmits *B. burgdorferi* in the western United States. These ticks are distinguished by their dark color and small size (about 1 mm in diameter as nymphs, and only 2 to 3 mm in diameter as unfed adults) (see Fig. 1.3). Other features include a distinct reddish coloration of the dorsum of the body of the adult female tick and black legs. Larval-stage ticks have six legs, and the nymphal- and adult-stage ticks have eight legs (Box 1.1).

A closely related species, *I. ricinus*, is the principal vector in western and central Europe (41–45), and *I. persulcatus* is the main vector in central and eastern Russia (52), China, and Japan (50). *I. ricinus* and *I. persulcatus*

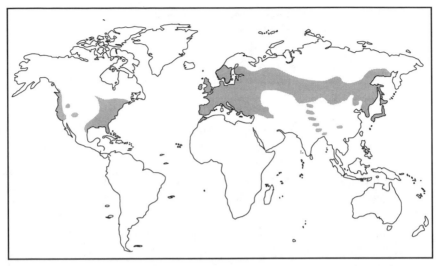

Figure 1.4   The global distribution of *Ixodes ricinus* species complex ticks able to transmit the Lyme disease spirochete. These ticks are found throughout temperate North America, Europe, and Asia. The principal vector in North America is *I. scapularis*, the black-legged (deer) tick. The principal vector in Europe is *I. ricinus*, and in Russia and northern Asia it is *I. persulcatus*. Each of these closely related vectors of Lyme disease can potentially transmit several other infectious agents, including human ehrlichioses, babesiosis, and encephalitis viruses. (Modified from Filippova NA, ed. Taiga tick, *Ixodes persulcatus* Schultze (Acarina, Ixodidae). Leningrad: Nauka Publishers; 1985.)

coexist in some areas of eastern Europe, and both tick species transmit the tick-borne encephalitis virus to humans.

Suspected cases of Lyme disease have been reported from sub-Saharan Africa, South America, and Australia, but no transmission cycles of *B. burgdorferi* have been identified at these sites, and no isolations of the Lyme disease spirochete have been made from suspected cases. In Canada, Lyme disease is believed to be endemic only in southeastern Ontario (53), although *I. scapularis* is found in limited foci elsewhere in eastern Canada and *I. pacificus* infected with *B. burgdorferi* has been found in British Columbia (54).

In the United States, rates of reported human infection by region are crudely related to rates of *B. burgdorferi* infection in vector ticks. Spirochete infection rates in nymphal and adult ticks are often 30% to 50% in highly endemic areas of the northeastern and mid-Atlantic regions and are generally 10% to 20% in the northcentral region. In contrast, these rates are only 1% to 2% in the Pacific coastal region and 0% to 3% in southeastern and southcentral states (41). The low infection rates of *Ixodes* vectors in the southern and western regions may be partly explained by the preferential feeding of immature-stage ticks on lizards in these regions. Lizards are incompetent reservoirs of *B. burgdorferi* and thus act as zooprophylactic hosts (41,55).

Box 1.1   Visual Identification of Deer Ticks

Season

- Nymphs feed from early May to August
- Adults feed from fall to early spring

Size

- Nymphs are typically 1 mm (poppy seed–sized)
- Unfed adults are 2–3 mm (sesame seed–sized)
  (An adult dog tick, for comparison, is two to four times larger than unfed adult deer tick)
- Engorged deer ticks may be as large as dog ticks

Markings/coloration

- Nymph is dark, dot-sized, has eight legs
- Adult is brown or black with orange-red crescent on dorsal shield, has eight black legs
  (An adult dog tick, for comparison, has prominent tan shield or brown spots, eight legs)

Environmental Factors

The ticks that transmit Lyme disease require shade, high humidity in their microenvironment, and ready access to preferred vertebrate hosts (45). In the United States, *I. scapularis* is most often found in moist coastal or riverine areas. The northeastern coastal and island habitat is characterized by dense brush dominated by scrub oak, pine, and bayberry bush, and the inland northeastern and northcentral habitat by mixed deciduous succession forests with sapling understory.

A study of tick distribution on large suburban residential properties in Westchester County, New York, found infective black-legged (deer) ticks on 60% of properties, with the greatest tick densities occurring in wooded areas, followed by fringe habitat, and much lesser densities among ornamental shrubbery and on lawns (56). Leaf litter provides a particularly favorable microenvironment for ixodid ticks.

The habitat in southern Atlantic coastal areas is complex mixed deciduous-conifer woodlands. *I. pacificus* in northern California is typically found in open oak woodland sites, where various tall grasses and chaparral are common ground cover (41). Geographic information systems data are being used to better define the various ecologic parameters associated with enzooticity and geographic spread (Box 1.2) (57,58).

Box 1.2   Prime Habitat for Lyme Disease Vectors

- High humidity environs (e.g., riverine, estuarial, and coastal habitat)
- Shaded, damp, forested, and brushy areas covered with leaf litter
- Especially areas frequented by deer: wood lots, wooded areas between yards, edges between yards and wooded or unmaintained brushy areas
- Areas frequented by mice and chipmunks (e.g., around woodpiles, stone walls, unkempt brushy areas, and tall grass at edges of residential properties)
- Brushy and grassy areas along hiking trails in areas frequented by deer
- Bayberry, scrub oak, and other scrub habitat in northeastern coastal fringe areas
- Oak-woodland and chaparral ground cover habitats of coastal northern California

---

Possible Alternate Arthropod Vectors of Infection

The lone star tick, *Amblyomma americanum*, has been suggested as a potential vector of the Lyme disease spirochete (59). The lone star tick is, however, an incompetent experimental vector of *B. burgdorferi* (60,61) and has not been found to play a role in maintaining a cycle of the Lyme disease spirochete in nature.

Spirochetes believed to be *B. burgdorferi* have been identified in blood-sucking insects, such as fleas, mosquitoes, and horseflies, but there is no indication that the organism is adapted for survival in these insects or that insects play any role in the maintenance of infection in nature. If blood-sucking arthropods other than ticks do sometimes mechanically transmit *B. burgdorferi*, such occurrences are likely to be rare and of little epidemiologic importance.

Vertebrate Hosts of Ticks and Spirochetes

The cycle of transmission of *B. burgdorferi* in the northeastern and mid-Atlantic coastal habitat is the most efficient and best-studied model of enzootic Lyme disease in the United States (43,62). In this model, the white-footed mouse is the most competent vertebrate reservoir (amplifying host) of *B. burgdorferi*. The mouse attains infection rates of 80% or more in highly endemic foci, maintains infection without apparent ill effects, and serves as the preferred vertebrate host for tick vectors in the immature stages. The chipmunk is also a highly competent reservoir host in the eastern United States.

Deer are incompetent reservoir hosts but appear to be a prerequisite for the establishment of black-legged tick populations (63). The explosive repopulation of the eastern United States by white-tailed deer in recent decades preceded the emergence of *I. scapularis* ticks and Lyme disease in this region. Wherever *I. scapularis* is found in large numbers, deer are numerous as well. However, *I. scapularis* is found on at least 33 species of mammals and 49

Table 1.1   Major Vertebrate Reservoirs of *Borrelia burgdorferi*

Eastern and Upper Northcentral U.S.*	West Coastal U.S.	Southern U.S.	Europe and Asia
White-footed mouse (*Peromyscus leucopus*)	Wood (pack) rat (*Neotoma* spp)	Cotton mouse	Voles (mostly)
Chipmunks	Kangaroo rat	Cotton rat	Various field and wood mice
Some ground-feeding birds	Deer mouse (*Peromyscus maniculatus*)	White-footed mouse	
Dogs		Raccoon	

*These animals also serve as principal sources of blood meals for immature-stage ticks (larvae, nymphs) of the black-legged tick that is a vector of Lyme disease.

species of birds (64), and the experimental removal of deer from selected areas results in the reduction, but not the elimination, of this tick in these areas (65). Alternate but less favorable tick maintenance hosts include raccoons, skunks, canids, and other medium- and large-sized mammals (Table 1.1).

Several bird species serve as maintenance hosts for vector ticks, and some species may serve as lesser reservoir hosts of *B. burgdorferi*. It is probable that migrating birds transport infected ticks that could then establish new enzootic foci (66). The Atlantic coastal strip, from Canada to Florida, is a major flyway, and birds may partly account for the rapid extension from the first described enzootic foci of *B. burgdorferi* in New England and Long Island, New York. Contiguous spread arising from the movement of deer and carnivores is most probably the principal factor in geographic spread of vector ticks.

Studies mapping the distribution of ticks, reservoir rodent hosts, and the seropositivity of dogs and deer and the incidence of human cases over time provide valuable information on the spread of Lyme disease in the United States (67,68). The seropositivity of dogs appears to be a sensitive and reliable epidemiologic marker of the geographic distribution of *B. burgdorferi* (69,70). Dogs have also recently been described as potential reservoirs of *B. burgdorferi* in the periresidential environment (71).

Epidemiology of Lyme Disease

Surveillance Statistics for the United States

Lyme disease was made a nationally notifiable disease in 1990. A uniform national case definition was adopted for surveillance purposes in 1991 (72), and reporting is now mandatory in all 50 states. Lyme disease accounts for

Table 1.2   Annual Totals Cases of Lyme Disease Reported by States to the Centers for Disease Control and Prevention, United States, 1991–1995

State	1991	1992	1993	1994	1995	Total
Alabama	13	10	4	6	12	45
Alaska	0	0	0	0	0	0
Arizona	1	0	0	0	1	2
Arkansas	31	20	8	15	11	85
California	265	231	134	68	84	782
Colorado	1	0	0	1	0	2
Connecticut	**1192**	**1760**	**1350**	**2030**	**1548**	**7880**
Delaware	73	219	143	106	56	597
District of Columbia	5	3	2	9	3	22
Florida	35	24	30	28	17	134
Georgia	25	48	44	127	14	258
Hawaii	0	2	1	0	0	3
Idaho	2	2	2	3	0	9
Illinois	51	41	19	24	18	153
Indiana	16	22	32	19	19	108
Iowa	22	33	8	17	16	96
Kansas	22	18	54	17	23	134
Kentucky	44	28	16	24	16	128
Louisiana	6	7	3	4	9	29
Maine	15	16	18	33	45	127
Maryland	**282**	**183**	**180**	**341**	**454**	**1440**
Massachusetts	**265**	**223**	**148**	**247**	**189**	**1072**
Michigan	46	35	23	33	5	142
Minnesota	**84**	**197**	**141**	**208**	**208**	**838**
Mississippi	8	0	0	0	17	25
Missouri	207	150	108	102	53	620
Montana	0	0	0	0	0	0
Nebraska	25	22	6	3	6	62
Nevada	5	1	5	1	6	18

Continued.

Table 1.2   Annual Totals Cases of Lyme Disease Reported by States to the Centers for Disease Control and Prevention, United States, 1991–1995—cont'd

State	1991	1992	1993	1994	1995	Total
New Hampshire	38	44	15	30	28	155
New Jersey	**915**	**688**	**786**	**1533**	**1703**	**5625**
New Mexico	3	2	2	5	1	13
New York	**3944**	**3448**	**2818**	**5200**	**4438**	**19,848**
North Carolina	73	67	86	77	84	387
North Dakota	2	1	2	0	0	5
Ohio	112	32	30	45	30	249
Oklahoma	29	27	19	99	63	237
Oregon	5	13	8	6	20	52
Pennsylvania	**718**	**1173**	**1085**	**1438**	**1562**	**5976**
Rhode Island	142	275	272	471	345	1,505
South Carolina	10	2	9	7	17	45
South Dakota	1	1	0	0	0	2
Tennessee	35	31	20	13	28	127
Texas	57	113	48	56	77	351
Utah	2	6	2	3	1	14
Vermont	7	9	12	16	9	53
Virginia	151	123	95	131	55	555
Washington	7	14	9	4	10	44
West Virginia	43	14	50	29	26	162
Wisconsin	**424**	**525**	**401**	**409**	**369**	**2128**
Wyoming	11	5	9	5	4	34
U.S. Total	**9470**	**9908**	**8257**	**13,043**	**11,700**	**52,378**

more than 90% of all reports of vector-borne infectious disease in the United States.

A provisional total of 11,603 cases of Lyme disease was reported by 43 states in 1995, compared with 497 cases by 11 states in 1982 (Table 1.2) (73). The national incidence of reported cases was 4.4 per 100,000 persons

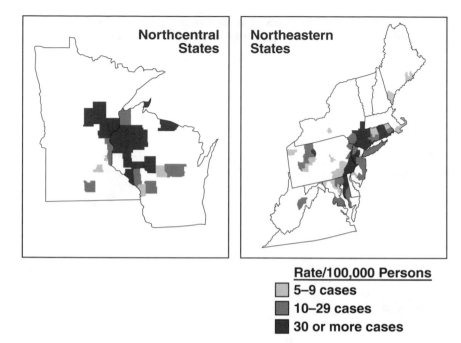

Figure 1.5   Rates of reported cases of Lyme disease, by county, in the endemic northeastern and northcentral regions of the United States during 1995. (Excludes counties with rates less than 5 cases per 100,000 persons.) Several counties in northwestern California also reported rates of more than 10 per 100,000 persons. Nationwide, 63 counties, each reporting 20 or more cases, accounted for 78% of all reported cases.

in 1995, ranging from 0 in several western states and Hawaii to 45.6 per 100,000 persons in Connecticut.

Geographic Distribution
The distribution of rates by county clearly shows geographic concentrations in the northeastern and northcentral regions (Fig. 1.5). Incidences of greater than 4.4 per 100,000 persons were reported by only eight states (Table 1.3), with these states accounting for more than 90% of the total number of reported cases. New York State alone accounts for more than 35% of reported cases, mostly from Suffolk and Westchester counties.

Clustering of cases by county, by township, and even by neighborhood is highly correlated with the abundance of vector ticks in the environment. Persons at greatest risk are residents of rural or suburban properties that are wooded or contiguous with wooded tracts inhabited by deer; others at relatively high risk include persons who live and vacation in northeastern coastal areas and in northcentral woodlands. Recent find-

Table 1.3   States with the Highest Rates of Reported Lyme Disease, 1995*

State	Rate/100,000 Persons	Number of Cases
Connecticut	45.6	1493
Rhode Island	34.9	345
New York	21.9	3978
New Jersey	21.1	1676
Pennsylvania	16.8	2018
Maryland	9.2	465
Wisconsin	7.2	369
Minnesota	5.8	269

*Provisional numbers at time of publication. Data from Centers for Disease Control and Prevention. Lyme disease: United States, 1995. MMWR Morb Mortal Wkly Rep. 1996;45:481-4.

ings of *I. scapularis* in deer-inhabited parks in greater New York City, Baltimore, and Philadelphia suggest the potential for a small but emerging urban risk.

Demographic Distribution
Lyme disease affects persons in all age groups, but the highest rates occur in children younger than 15 years of age and in adults 30 years of age and older (Fig. 1.6). Males and females are nearly equally affected. National surveillance data for 1995 provide the following demographic breakdown: males, 51%; 0 to 14 years old, 24%; 35 to 49 years old, 24%; white, 95.8%; black 2.4%; other race, 1.8% (73).

Flaws with Case Reporting
Lyme disease case reporting is fraught with problems of misclassification, misdiagnosis, and under-reporting. From 1991 to 1992 in Connecticut, more than 80% of all cases of Lyme disease in the state registry were reported by physicians from four primary care specialties, but only 7% of physicians in these specialties had reported cases (74). Follow-up interviews with a sample of physicians in the four specialty areas suggested that less than 20% of all cases diagnosed and treated as incident cases of Lyme disease had been reported. A recent study in Maryland suggested that Lyme disease is under-reported by 10- to 12-fold in that state and that many more patients are seen and treated for presumptive Lyme disease and for tick bite alone than patients meeting the case criteria for reporting (75).

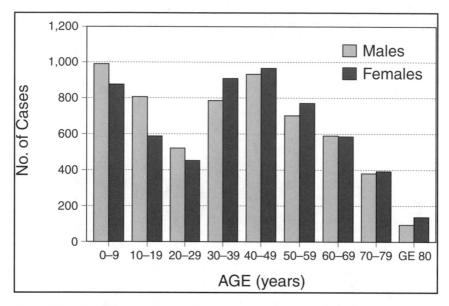

Figure 1.6   Rates of reported cases of Lyme disease by age and sex in the United States during 1995 (*n* = 11,700). Lyme disease affects persons in all age groups, but the highest rates occur among children younger than 15 years old and adults 30 years of age and older.

Lyme Disease Emergence

Lyme disease is one of several emerging tick-borne diseases in the United States (40,76). Since 1980 several outbreaks of Lyme disease have been described in the eastern localities, which provide important information on the emergence of the disease in populations newly at risk under differing epidemiologic circumstances (77).

Residence in new suburban housing developments, and occupational exposures among outdoor workers at a military reservation were shown to be risk factors in two New Jersey studies (78,79). A study on Fire Island, a barrier island off the south coast of Long Island, New York, described a cumulative prevalence of 7.5% and a seasonal incidence of 1% to 3% among residents of this summer vacation site (33). A longitudinal study of a community of approximately 160 persons on Great Island, Massachusetts, found a slow build-up of incidence to a peak of 3% per year and a total cumulative prevalence of 16% over a 20-year period (34).

A similar restricted population in the northern coastal area of Ipswich, Massachusetts, experienced an outbreak of Lyme disease during the 1980s (27). The attack rate from 1980 through 1987 was 35% among 190 residents living within 5 km of a nature preserve heavily infested with *B. burgdor-*

feri–infected ticks; the annual incidence reached a peak of 10%, and several residents became reinfected one or more times. Population-based studies in highly endemic suburban communities in northern Westchester County, New York, described a seasonal attack rate of 2.6% and a prevalence of 8.8% (80).

The introduction and build-up of Lyme disease to highly endemic levels within some states and regions over the past two decades is a considerable public health concern, especially because no practical strategy has been developed to prevent its enzootic spread. The build-up has been most pronounced in suburban and rural residential areas in northeastern states. A review of surveillance data in Connecticut for the period of 1977 to 1985 suggests a threefold to eightfold increase in incidence in the communities originally studied by Steere and colleagues during the mid-1970s (4) and an extension of disease from one county to all counties within the state (81).

Rapid emergence has also been well documented in New York State (82). Before 1979, vector ticks were known to be present only in eastern Long Island, but by 1989, they were recognized in 22 New York counties, and enzootic cycles of *B. burgdorferi* were described in eight adjacent counties in southern New York. The Hudson River Valley appears to be a natural avenue of spread, and the latest count identifies 34 New York counties where *I. scapularis* has been found, including counties bordering on Canada.

Endemic Lyme disease extends from southern Maine to Maryland, whereas enzootic cycles of *B. burgdorferi* of undetermined public health importance extend further along the southern Atlantic Coast to northern Florida, with greatest enzootic intensity occurring on barrier islands. Patterns of disease emergence similar to those in New York have been noted in New Jersey (79) and in Wisconsin (83,84). Enzootic *B. burgdorferi* is found in areas of Minnesota, Illinois, and northern Michigan that are contiguous with known foci in Wisconsin.

Lyme disease appears to be more stable in the Pacific coastal region, where the majority of reported human cases occur in a few counties in northern California.

Areas with Unconfirmed Endemicity

The reporting of cases from areas where ticks are not known to transmit *B. burgdorferi* to humans, such as throughout many southern, midwestern, and mountain states, remains enigmatic. In the southern United States, *I. scapularis* is an inefficient vector of *B. burgdorferi* and rarely feeds on humans. Epidemiologic studies in Missouri of persons with EM-like lesions and of area-matched controls provide evidence that the disease in this area is associated with tick bites but is not caused by *B. burgdorferi* or other known tick-borne infection (85).

Box 1.3   Major Risk Factors for Acquiring Lyme Disease

Residence in an endemic residential community:

- Wooded suburban and rural areas of coastal New England and mid-Atlantic states
- Wooded areas of Wisconsin and Minnesota
- Some northern coastal California counties (lesser risk)
- Properties on which deer are regularly seen in these areas (highest risk)
  Gardening, brush-clearing, and outdoor recreation are individual risk factors in these environments.

Vacation stays or spring/summer outdoor-recreational activities in endemic areas:

- Natural environments of coastal New England and mid-Atlantic states
- Wooded areas of Wisconsin and Minnesota

Occupational exposures in tick-infested environments:

Any of the following occupations are risk factors in these environments:
- Landscaper
- Right-of-way clearing crew member
- Forester
- Surveyor

EM-like lesions were noted in this study (85) and by others to occur after bites by the lone star tick, *Amblyomma americanum*. The lone star tick is widely distributed throughout the southern and mid-Atlantic regions, and it is the most common human-biting tick in the South. Recent studies using polymerase chain reaction techniques have identified a new, uncultivable spirochete, *Borrelia lonestari* sp. nov., in darkfield-positive *A. americanum* (86), but there is no proof as yet that *B. lonestari* causes infection in humans.

Risk Factors for Infection with the Lyme Disease Spirochete

Lyme disease is a disease of place. The principal risk factor for Lyme disease in the United States is permanent or seasonal residence in an endemic area (i.e., an area with high infestation with infected ticks) (Box 1.3). Endemic areas include the following:

- Coastal fringe and island areas of New England
- Selected wooded residential communities and natural areas of the northeastern states, mainly from Massachusetts to Maryland

- Rural wooded areas of Wisconsin, northern Michigan, eastern Minnesota, and selected counties of northwestern California

Exposures to infected ticks are most likely in the parts of residential properties and surroundings that are relatively undisturbed—for example, tall grass, brushy scrub, and wooded tracts. Recreational activities in natural areas, such as hiking, camping, fishing, and hunting, also expose persons to infected ticks, especially during the late spring and summer months. Outdoor occupations, such as landscaping, surveying, brush clearing, forestry, and wildlife and parks management, may place persons at high risk in some areas.

A study of employees in New Jersey showed that outdoor workers were more than four times as likely to have had Lyme disease as indoor workers (78). A comprehensive study of workers in endemic counties of downstate New York showed that persons with a history of outdoor employment were twice as likely to be seropositive as those without such a history (87). Although the difference was not statistically significant, in a separate comparison, the seroprevalence rate of outdoor employees was 5.9 times higher than that of a comparison group of anonymous blood donors from the same region of New York. However, the most important risk factor for Lyme disease among New York workers was a history of spending 30 or more hours of leisure per week outdoors, an association that was not found in some other studies (33,88). Studies in Europe have shown occupational risks associated with forestry, and serologic evidence of high *B. burgdorferi* exposure in forest workers was positively associated with a worker's age, history of tick bite, and history of EM (89,90).

In early studies in Connecticut (88), ownership of cats was found to be associated with an increased risk of acquiring Lyme disease, and domestic cats were observed to bring unattached nymphal ticks into homes in an endemic area of New York (where 49% of nymphal ticks collected from vegetation were found to be infected with *B. burgdorferi*) (91). A study of dogs and persons living in the same households in two highly endemic areas in Massachusetts showed that dogs were more likely to have serologic evidence of *B. burgdorferi* infection than their human co-residents; furthermore, although methods of selection of controls were not described, the authors noted that there was no difference in the risk of infection between people from the dog-owning households and other residents in the study sites (70).

Prevention

Avoidance and Personal Protection

The best means of preventing Lyme disease are avoidance of tick-infested areas, personal protection, environmental management, and early detection

---

Box 1.4   Protection Pointers for the Public

- Know tick-infested areas and avoid them. Stay out of unkempt brushy and grassy areas.
- When you are in a tick-infested environment, wear light-colored clothing and long sleeves, tuck pant-legs into socks, and apply insect repellents to exposed skin and clothing as directed. Inspect yourself and family members daily for ticks.
- Remove attached ticks promptly and correctly with tweezers.
- Know the signs and symptoms of early Lyme disease or other tick-borne infection (e.g., fever, headache, chills, body aches and pains, rash). See your doctor right away if you believe that you may have a tick-borne illness.
- Consider modifications to your residential landscape, such as clearing of leaf litter, brush, and tall grass; pruning of shrubs and trees to open up shaded areas to sunlight; removing stone walls and woodpiles; erecting deer barriers.

---

and treatment of disease manifestations (Box 1.4). The public should be informed about which areas are known to be tick infested and about avoiding risky exposures, especially during the spring and summer. Information on the distribution of ticks in an area can usually be obtained from health departments and park or agricultural extension services.

When in tick-infested areas, persons should wear light-colored clothing so that ticks on clothing can be spotted more easily and removed. Persons should also wear long-sleeved shirts and tuck pants into socks or boot tops to prevent ready access of ticks to skin. Ticks, especially nymphs and larvae, quest close to the ground, and entomologists who work in tick-infested areas find that wearing high rubber boots prevents tick attachment; this is also a simple protection for persons clearing leaf litter and underbrush from wooded properties.

Insect repellents containing diethyltoluamide (DEET) can be applied to clothes and to exposed skin other than the face, and permethrin compounds (which kill ticks on contact) can be sprayed on clothing.

One of the most important preventive measures is the early detection and proper removal of skin-attached ticks. Tweezers should be used to grasp the tick mouthparts, and the tick removed by steady, gentle traction. Studies have shown that transmission of *B. burgdorferi* from an infected tick is unlikely to occur before 48 hours of attachment (92). When persons are in tick-infested areas, a daily check for ticks and their proper removal are important measures for preventing infection.

Antibiotic treatment (prophylaxis) to prevent Lyme disease after a known tick bite is not routinely warranted. The risk of asymptomatic infection or disease in untreated persons has been found to be less than 3%, even when they are bitten by known vector species in highly endemic areas. This risk of exposure is, in most circumstances, below the cost–benefit threshold of treatment (93,94).

Landscape Management and Tick Control

In endemic residential areas of the northeastern United States, wood lots, stone fences, and unkempt edges of yards pose a significantly greater risk than lawns and ornamental shrubby areas (56). Removing leaf litter and woodpiles and clearing trees and brush around houses and at the edges of yards to admit more sunlight and remove habitat suitable for deer, ticks, and rodent reservoirs of infection may reduce the numbers of ticks that transmit Lyme disease in the ensuing transmission seasons.

Area application of acaricides to residential properties has been found to be highly effective in suppressing vector ticks but raises environmental concerns (95,96). The distribution in yards of acaricide-impregnated cotton balls, which mice then use for nest building, has produced variable results (45,97,98). Excluding deer from properties and maintaining tick-free pets may reduce tick numbers in the immediate periresidential environment (45,99).

No known practical measures exist for controlling tick vectors or rodent reservoirs of infection over large areas. Similarly, there are no means for effectively controlling rodent reservoirs of infection. Management of deer populations and control of ticks on deer would seem to be a logical strategy for reducing the intensity of enzootic transmission in already established foci of infection and for limiting spread to new areas. The control of ticks on deer using self-dosing systems for applying topical and systemic acaricides is being evaluated in pilot trials.

Vaccination

Vaccines against infection with *B. burgdorferi* have been developed for both dogs and humans (see also Chapter 10). Phase III trials of three-dose recombinant Osp-A immunization in humans, involving approximately 20,000 participants and using vaccines by two manufacturers, have recently been completed in endemic areas of the northcentral and northeastern United States. A unique aspect of the Osp-A vaccine is the killing of *B. burgdorferi* within the midgut of ticks feeding on immunized experimental animal hosts (100).

■   ■   ■

Key Points

- Lyme disease is a rapidly emerging zoonosis caused by the spirochete *Borrelia burgdorferi*, which is transmitted via a tick vector, *Ixodes scapularis* (in the eastern United States) or *I. pacificus* (in the western United States).

- More than 10,000 cases are reported yearly in the United States, with only eight states accounting for more than 90% of the total number of reported cases: Connecticut, Rhode Island, New York, New Jersey, Pennsylvania, Maryland, Wisconsin, and Minnesota.

- Risk is greatest in the spring and summer, when persons in endemic areas are most likely to be bitten by the small and easily overlooked nymphal-stage *Ixodes* ticks.

- Persons can reduce their risk by avoiding tick-infested habitats; using protective clothing, insect repellents, and insecticides; detecting attached ticks early and removing them properly; and removing harborage and food for rodents, deer, and ticks in their residential environment.

■ ■ ■

REFERENCES

1. **Hellerstrom S.** Erythema chronicum migrans Afzelius with meningitis. South Med J. 1950;43:330-5.

2. **Scrimenti RJ.** Erythema chronicum migrans. Arch Dermatol. 1970;102:104-5.

3. **Steere AC, Malawista SE, Hardin JA, et al.** Erythema chronicum migrans and Lyme arthritis: the enlarging clinical spectrum. Ann Intern Med. 1977;86:685-98.

4. **Steere AC, Malawista SE, Snydman DR, et al.** Lyme arthritis: an epidemic of oligoarticular arthritis in children and adults in three Connecticut communities. Arthritis Rheum. 1977;20:7-17.

5. **Steere AC, Malawista SE, Newman JH, et al.** Antibiotic therapy in Lyme disease. Ann Intern Med. 1980;93:1-8.

6. **Burgdorfer WA, Barbour AG, Hayes SF, et al.** Lyme disease: a tick-borne spirochetosis? Science. 1982;216:1317-9.

7. **Barbour AG.** Isolation and cultivation of Lyme disease spirochetes. Yale J Biol Med. 1984;57:521-5.

8. **Steere AC, Grodzicki RL, Kornblatt AN, et al.** The spirochetal etiology of Lyme disease. N Engl J Med. 1983;308:733-40.

9. **Benach JL, Bosler EM, Hanrahan JP, et al.** Spirochetes isolated from the blood of two patients with Lyme disease. N Engl J Med. 1983;308:740-2.

10. **Johnson RC, Schmid GP, Hyde FW, et al.** *Borrelia burgdorferi* sp. nov.: etiologic agent of Lyme disease. Int J Syst Bacteriol. 1984;34:496-7.

11. **Barbour AG, Hayes SF.** Biology of *Borrelia* species. Microbiol Rev. 1986;50:381-400.

12. **Rosa PA, Schwan TG.** Molecular biology of *Borrelia burgdorferi*. In: Coyle PK, ed. Lyme Disease. St. Louis: Mosby–Year Book; 1993:8-17.

13. **Adam T, Gossmann GS, Rasiah C, et al.** Phenotypic and genotypic analysis of *Borrelia burgdorferi* isolates from various sources. Infect Immun. 1991;59:2579-85.

14. **Jonsson M, Noppa L, Barbour AG.** Heterogeneity of outer membrane proteins in *Borrelia burgdorferi*: comparison of ospoperons of three isolates of different geographic origins. Infect Immun. 1992;60:1845-53.

15. **Baranton G, Postic D, Saint-Girons I, et al.** Delineation of *Borrelia burgdorferi* sensu stricto, *Borrelia garinii* sp. nov., and Group V5461 associated with Lyme borreliosis. Int J Syst Bacteriol. 1991;42:378-83.

16. **van Dam AP, Kuiper H, Vos K, et al.** Different genospecies of *Borrelia burgdorferi* are associated with distinct clinical manifestations of Lyme borreliosis. Clin Infect Dis. 1993;17:708-17.

17. **Anthonissen FM, De Kesel M, Hoet PP, Bigaignon GH.** Evidence for the involvement of different genospecies of *Borrelia* in the clinical outcome of Lyme disease in Belgium. Res Microbiol. 1994;145:327-31.

18. **Schlesinger PA, Duray PH, Burke PA, et al.** Maternal-fetal transmission of the Lyme disease spirochete, *Borrelia burgdorferi*. Ann Intern Med. 1985;103:67-8.

19. **Gerber MA, Shapiro ED, Krause PJ, et al.** The risk of acquiring Lyme disease or babesiosis from a blood transfusion. J Infect Dis. 1994;170:231-34.

20. **Steere AC.** Lyme disease. N Engl J Med. 1989;321:586-96.

21. **Berger BW, Johnson RC, Kodner C, et al.** Cultivation of *Borrelia burgdorferi* from erythema migrans lesions and perilesional skin. J Clin Microbiol. 1992;30:359-61.

22. **Berardi VP, Weeks KE, Steere AC.** Serodiagnosis of early Lyme disease: analysis of IgM and IgG antibody responses by using an antibody-capture enzyme immunoassay. J Infect Dis. 1988;158:754-60.

23. **Dressler F, Whalen JA, Reinhardt BN, et al.** Western immunoblotting in the serodiagnosis of Lyme disease. J Infect Dis. 1993;167:392-400.

24. **Johnson BJB, Robbins KE, Bailey RE, et al.** Serodiagnosis of Lyme disease: accuracy of a two-step approach using a flagella-based ELISA and immunoblotting. J Infect Dis. 1996;174:346-53.

25. **Dattwyler RJ, Volkman DJ, Luft BJ, et al.** Seronegative Lyme disease: dissociation of the specific T- and B-lymphocyte responses to *Borrelia burgdorferi*. N Engl J Med. 1988;319:1441-6.

26. **Logigian EL, Kaplan RF, Steere AC.** Chronic neurologic manifestations of Lyme disease. N Engl J Med. 1990;323:1438-44.

27. **Lastavica CC, Wilson M, Berardi VP, et al.** Rapid emergence of a focal epidemic of Lyme disease in coastal Massachusetts. N Engl J Med. 1989;320:133-7.

28. **Weber K, Schierz G, Wilske B, et al.** Reinfection with erythema migrans disease. Infection. 1986;14:32-5.

29. **Pfister HW, Preac-Mursic V, Wilske B, et al.** Randomized comparisons of ceftriaxone and cefotaxime in Lyme neuroborreliosis. J Infect Dis. 1991;163:311-8.

30. **Snydman DR, Schenkein DP, Berardi VP, et al.** *Borrelia burgdorferi* in joint fluid in chronic Lyme disease. Ann Intern Med. 1986;104:798-800.

31. **Stanek G, Klein J, Bittner R, et al.** Isolation of *Borrelia burgdorferi* from the myocardium of a patient with longstanding cardiomyopathy. N Engl J Med. 1990;322:249-52.

32. **Strle F, Cheng Y, Cimperman J, et al.** Persistence of *Borrelia burgdorferi* sensu lato in resolved erythema migrans lesions. Clin Infect Dis. 1995;21:380-9.

33. **Hanrahan JP, Benach JL, Coleman JL, et al.** Incidence and cumulative frequency of Lyme disease in a community. J Infect Dis. 1984;150:489-96.

34. **Steere AC, Taylor E, Wilson ML, et al.** Longitudinal assessment of the clinical and epidemiologic features of Lyme disease in a defined population. J Infect Dis. 1986;154:295-300.

35. **Steere AC, Dwyer E, Winchester R.** Association of chronic Lyme arthritis with HLA-DR4 and HLA-DR2 alleles. N Engl J Med. 1990;323:219-23.

36. **Markowitz LE, Steere AC, Benach JL, et al.** Lyme disease during pregnancy. JAMA. 1986;255:3394-6.

37. **Williams CL, Strobino B, Weinstein A, et al.** Maternal Lyme disease and congenital malformations: a cord blood serosurvey in endemic and control areas. Paediatr Perinat Epidemiol. 1995;9:320-30.

38. **Krause PJ, Telford SR, Spielman A, et al.** Concurrent Lyme disease and babesiosis: evidence for increased severity and duration of illness. JAMA. 1996;275:1657-60.

39. **Marcus LC, Steere AC, Duray PH, et al.** Fatal pancarditis in a patient with coexistent Lyme disease and babesiosis. Ann Intern Med. 1985;103:374-6.

40. **Fishbein DB, Dennis DT.** Tick-borne diseases: a growing risk. N Engl J Med. 1995;333:452-3.

41. **Lane RS, Piesman J, Burgdorfer W.** Lyme borreliosis: relation of its causative agent to its vectors and hosts in North America and Europe. Annu Rev Entomol. 1991;36:587-609.

42. **Hashimoto Y, Kawagishi N, Sakai H, et al.** Lyme disease in Japan. Analysis of *Borrelia* species using rRNA gene restriction fragment length polymorphism. Dermatology. 1995;191:193-8.

43. **Spielman A, Wilson ML, Levine JF, et al.** Ecology of *Ixodes dammini*-borne human babesiosis and Lyme disease. Annu Rev Entomol. 1985;30:439-460.

44. **Telford SR III, Mather TN, Moore SI, et al.** Incompetence of deer as reservoirs of the Lyme disease spiro chete. Am J Trop Med Hyg. 1988;39:105-9.

45. **Piesman J, Gray JS.** Lyme disease/Lyme borreliosis. In: Sonenshine DE, Mather TN, eds. Ecological Dynamics of Tick-Borne Zoonoses. New York: Oxford University Press; 1994:327-50.

46. **Dekonenko EJ, Steere AC, Berardi VP, Kravchuk LN.** Lyme borreliosis in the Soviet Union: a cooperative US-USSR report. J Infect Dis. 1988;158:748-53.

47. **Miyamoto K, Nakao M, Uchikawa K, et al.** Prevalence of Lyme borreliosis spirochetes in ixodid ticks of Japan, with special reference to a new potential vector, *Ixodes ovatus* (Acari:Ixodidae). J Med Entomol. 1992;29:216-20.

48. **Schmid GP.** The global distribution of Lyme disease. Rev Infect Dis. 1985;7:41-50.

49. **Ai CX, Hu RJ, Hyland KE, et al.** Epidemiological and aetiological evidence for the transmission of Lyme disease by adult *Ixodes persulcatus* in an endemic area in China. Inter J Epidemiol. 1990;19:1061-5.

50. **Carlberg H, Naito S.** Lyme borreliosis: a review and present situation in Japan. J Dermatol. 1991;18:125-42.

51. **Berglund J, Eitrem R, Ornstein K, et al.** An epidemiologic study of Lyme disease in southern Sweden. N Engl J Med. 1995;333:1319-24.

52. **Kornberg EI, Kovalevsky YV, Kryuchechnikov VN, Gorelova NB.** Tick *Ixodes* persulcatus Schulze, 1930 as a vector of *Borrelia burgdorferi*. In: F Dusbabek, V Bukva, eds. Modern Acarology. Prague: Academia; 1991;1:119-23.

53. Lyme disease in Canada. Can Dis Wkly Rep. 1990;16:141-52.

54. **Banerjee SN.** Isolation of *Borrelia burgdorferi* in British Columbia. Can Commun Dis Rep. 1993;19:204-05.

55. **Spielman A, Levine JF, Wilson ML.** Vectorial capacity of North American *Ixodes* ticks. Yale J Biol Med. 1994;57:507-13.

56. **Maupin GO, Fish D, Zultowsky J, et al.** Landscape ecology of Lyme disease in a residential area of Westchester County, New York. Am J Epidemiol. 1991;133:1105-13.

57. **Glass GE, Amerisinghe FP, Morgan JM, et al.** Predicting *Ixodes scapularis* abundance on white-tailed deer using geographic information systems. Am J Trop Med Hyg. 1994;51:538-44.

58. **Kitron U, Jones CJ, Bouseman JK, et al.** Spatial analysis of the distribution of *Ixodes dammini* (Acari: Ixodidae) on white-tailed deer in Ogle County, Illinois. J Med Entomol. 1992;29:259-66.

59. **Schulze TL, Bowen GS, Bosler EM, et al.** *Amblyomma americanum*: a potential vector of Lyme disease in New Jersey. Science. 1984;224:601-3.

60. **Mukolwe SW, Kocan AA, Barker RW, et al.** Attempted transmission of *Borrelia burgdorferi* (Spirochaetales: Spirochaetaceae) (JDI Strain) by *Ixodes scapularis* (Acari: Ixodidae), *Dermacentor variabilis,* and *Amblyomma americanum.* J Med Entomol. 1992;29:673-7.

61. **Piesman J, Sinsky RJ.** Ability of *Ixodes scapularis, Dermacentor variabilis,* and *Amblyomma americanum* (Acari:Ixodidae) to acquire, maintain, and transmit Lyme disease spirochetes (*Borrelia burgdorferi*). J Med Entomol. 1988;25:336-9.

62. **Spielman A.** Human babesiosis on Nantucket Island: transmission by nymphal *Ixodes* ticks. Am J Trop Med Hyg. 1976;25.784-7.

63. **Wilson ML, Adler GH, Spielman A.** Correlation between abundance of deer and that of the deer tick, *Ixodes dammini* (Acari: Ixodidae). Ann Entomol Soc Am. 1985;78:172-6.

64. **Anderson JF.** Mammalian and avian reservoirs for *Borrelia burgdorferi.* Ann N Y Acad Sci. 1985;539:180-91.

65. **Wilson ML, Telford SR, III, Piesman J, et al.** Reduced abundance of immature *Ixodes dammini* (Acari:Ixodidae) following elimination of deer. J Med Entomol. 1988;25:224-8.

66. **Anderson JF.** Epizootiology of *Borrelia* in tick vectors and reservoir hosts. Rev Infect Dis. 1989;11:S1451-8.

67. **Lindenmayer JM, Marshall D, Onderdonk AB.** Dogs as sentinels for Lyme disease in Massachusetts. Am J Pub Health. 1991;81:1448-55.

68. **Rand PW, Smith RP, Lacombe EH.** Canine seroprevalence and the distribution of *Ixodes dammini* in an area of emerging Lyme disease. Am J Pub Health. 1991;81:1331-4.

69. **Daniels TJ, Fish D, Levine JF, et al.** Canine exposure to *Borrelia burgdorferi* and prevalence of *Ixodes dammini* (Acari:Ixodidae) on deer as a measure of Lyme disease risk in the northeastern United States. J Med Entomol. 1993;30:171-8.

70. **Eng TR, Wilson MI, Spielman A, et al.** Greater risk of *Borrelia burgdorferi* infection in dogs than people. J Infect Dis. 1988;158:1410-1.

71. **Mather TN, Fish D, Coughlin RT.** Competence of dogs as reservoirs for Lyme disease spirochetes (Borrelia burgdorferi). JAVMA. 1994;205:186-8.

72. **Centers for Disease Control and Prevention.** Case definitions for public health surveillance. MMWR. 1990;39(RR-13):19-21.

73. **Centers for Disease Control and Prevention.** Lyme disease: United States, 1995. MMWR. 1996;45:481-4.

74. **Centers for Disease Control and Prevention.** Physician reporting of Lyme disease: Connecticut, 1991–1992. MMWR. 1993;42:348-50.

75. **Coyle BS, Strickland GT, Liang YY, et al.** The public health impact of Lyme disease in Maryland. J Infect Dis. 1996;173:1260-2.

76. **Spach DH, Liles WC, Campbell GL, et al.** Tick-borne diseases in the United States. N Engl J Med. 1993;329:936-47.

77. **Dennis DT.** Lyme disease: tracking an epidemic (editorial). JAMA. 1991;266:1269-70.

78. **Bowen SG, Schultze TL, Hayne C, et al.** A focus of Lyme disease in Monmouth County, New Jersey. Am J Epidemiol. 1984;120:387-94.

79. **Schulze TL, Shisler JK, Bosler EM, et al.** Evolution of a focus of Lyme disease. Zentral l Bakteriol Hyg. 1986;A263:65-71.

80. **Alpert B, Esin J, Sivak SL, et al.** Incidence and prevalence of Lyme disease in a suburban Westchester County community. N Y State J Med. 1992;92:5-8.

81. **Cartter ML, Mshar P, Hadler JL.** The epidemiology of Lyme disease in Connecticut. Conn Med. 1989;53:320-3.

82. **White DJ, Chang H-G, Benach JL, et al.** The geographic spread and temporal increase of the Lyme disease epidemic. JAMA. 1991;266:1230-6.

83. **Davis JP, Schell WL, Amundson TE, et al.** Lyme disease in Wisconsin: epidemiologic, clinical, serologic, and entomologic findings. Yale J Biol Med. 1984;57:685-96.

84. **French JB, Jr, Schell WL, Kazmierczak JJ, et al.** Changes in population density and distribution of *Ixodes dammini* (Acari:Ixodidae) in Wisconsin during the 1980s. J Med Entomol. 1992;29:723-8.

85. **Campbell GL, Paul WS, Schriefer ME, et al.** Epidemiologic and diagnostic studies of patients with suspected early Lyme disease, Missouri. J Infect Dis. 1995; 172:470-80.

86. **Barbour AG, Maupin GO, Teltow GJ, et al.** An uncultivable *Borrelia* sp. in the hard tick, *Amblyomma americanum:* a possible agent of a Lyme disease–like disease. J Infect Dis. 1996;173:403-9.

87. **Smith PF, Benach JL, White DJ, et al.** Occupational risk of Lyme disease in endemic areas of New York State. Ann N Y Acad Sci. 1988;539:289-301.

88. **Steere AC, Broderick TF, Malawista SE.** Erythemachronicum migrans and Lyme arthritis: epidemiologic evidence for a tick vector. Am J Epidemiol. 1978;108:312-21.

89. **Kuiper H, deJongh BM, Nauta AP, et al.** Lyme borreliosis in Dutch forestry workers. J Infect. 1991;23:279-86.

90. **Neubert U, Munchhoff P, Volker B, et al.** *Borrelia burgdorferi* infections in Bavarian forest workers. Ann N Y Acad Sci. 1988;539:476-9.

91. **Curran KL, Fish D.** Increased risk of Lyme disease for cat owners (letter). N Engl J Med. 1989;320:183.

92. **Piesman J, Maupin GO, Campos EG, et al.** Duration of adult female *Ixodes dammini* attachment and transmission of *Borrelia burgdorferi,* with description of a needle aspiration isolation method. J Infect Dis. 1991;163:895-7.

93. **Shapiro ED, Gerber MA, Holabird NB, et al.** A controlled trial of antimicrobial prophylaxis for Lyme disease after deer-tick bites. N Engl J Med. 1992;327:1769-73.

94. **Magid D, Schwartz B, Craft J, Schwartz JS.** Prevention of Lyme disease after tick bites: a cost-effectiveness analysis. N Eng J Med. 1992;327:534-41.

95. **Curran KL, Fish D, Piesman J.** Reduction of nymphal *Ixodes dammini* (Acari:Ixodidae) in a residential suburban landscape by area application of insecticides. J Med Entomol. 1993;30:107-13.

96. **Schultze TL, Jordan RA, Vasvary LM, et al.** Suppression of *Ixodes scapularis* (Acarai:Ixodidae) nymphs in a large residential community. J Med Entomol. 1994; 31:206-11.

97. **Stafford KC III.** Effectiveness of host-targeted permethrin in the control of *Ixodes dammini* (Acari:Ixodidae). J Med Entomol. 1991;28:611-7.

98. **Mather TN, Ribiero JM, Moore SI, et al.** Reducing transmission of Lyme disease in a suburban setting. Ann N Y Acad Med. 1988;539:402-3.

99. **Daniels TJ, Fish D, Schwartz I.** Reduced abundance of *Ixodes scapularis* (Acari·Ixodidae) and Lyme disease risk by deer exclusion. J Med Entomol. 1993;30:1043-9.

100. **Telford SR, Fikrig E, Barthold SW, et al.** Protection against antigenically variable *Borrelia burgdorferi* conferred by recombinant vaccines. J Exp Med. 1993;178:755-8.

KEY REFERENCES

Centers for Disease Control and Prevention. Lyme disease: United States, 1996. MMWR. 1997;46:531-5.

Annual update on the national surveillance statistics on Lyme disease in the United States. The data reinforce previous observations that Lyme disease is highly localized to a few states in the northeastern and upper northcentral regions. Connecticut, Rhode Island, New York, New Jersey, Pennsylvania, Delaware, Maryland, and Wisconsin alone accounted for 91% of the 16,535 cases reported in 1996.

Coyle BS, Strickland GT, Liang YY, et al. The public health impact of Lyme disease in Maryland. J Infect Dis. 1996;173:1260-2.

This study estimates the health burden imposed by Lyme disease in Maryland. A 1-in-15 survey of physicians was used to estimate the numbers of cases of diagnosed Lyme disease, presumptive Lyme disease, patients with tick bites, and diagnostic tests ordered for Lyme disease. Results indicated that Lyme disease was under-reported by 10- to 12-fold in Maryland; that 80% of cases were managed by primary care physicians; and that because of overdiagnosis, nearly five times as many patients who did not have Lyme disease were treated for the condition or for tick bite than patients meeting standard clinical and serologic criteria for Lyme disease.

Speilman A. The emergence of Lyme disease and babesiosis in a changing environment. Ann N Y Acad Sci. 1994;740:146-56.

A thoughtful review of the emergence of human Lyme disease and babesiosis in the United States and Europe, the epizootiology of these diseases, and the principal factors underlying their emergence (in particular the reforestation of the eastern United States and the consequent explosion of deer and deer tick populations).

Steere AC, Taylor E, Wilson ML, et al. Longitudinal assessment of the clinical and epidemiological features of Lyme disease in a defined population. J Infect Dis. 1986; 154:295-300.

Describes the evolution of highly endemic Lyme disease in a coastal Massachusetts community (Great Island, Massachusetts), defining the incidence and cumulative prevalence of illness as well as the incidence and persistence of antibodies to B. burgdorferi *in the serum of affected residents.*

2

■ ■ ■

Natural History of Lyme Disease

Daniel W. Rahn, MD

Knowledge about Lyme disease has expanded dramatically since the original description of the disease in 1975, but so have the areas of uncertainty and the public and professional misconceptions about this complex illness. In this chapter, the natural history of *untreated* Lyme disease is reviewed, dispelling some of the myths about what constitutes typical Lyme disease and with special emphasis on the common clinical manifestations and the usual disease course. The information presented in this chapter is based on solid clinical evidence, with reference to areas of current controversy or uncertainty. The complete range of specific organ system manifestations and response to treatment are discussed in other chapters in this text.

The typical clinical features of each stage of Lyme disease and the usual time course and serologic response of each stage are presented in Figure 2.1. Although the disease course itself is highly variable, the progression from acute, episodic inflammation to chronic inflammation does not vary.

Early Localized Lyme Disease

Lyme disease typically begins with the characteristic (but not pathognomonic) skin lesion erythema migrans (EM) at the site of a bite by an infected tick. The name of this lesion has been shortened from erythema chronicum migrans because, for most persons, this skin lesion is not chronic. Erythema migrans begins as a small papule or macule at the site of a bite by an infected tick (1).

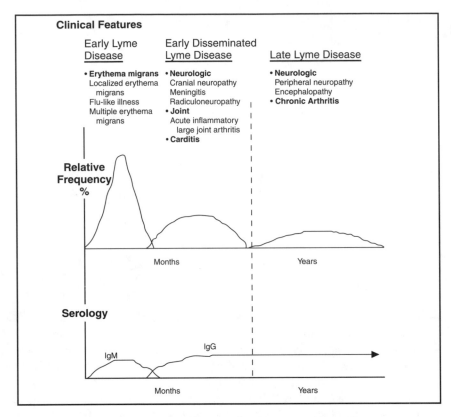

Figure 2.1   Natural history of serologic response in untreated Lyme disease.

Tick Bite and Transmission of Infection

Transmission of infection does not occur as readily as is commonly thought. Several factors determine the likelihood that a tick bite will result in Lyme disease. Even in highly endemic areas, only a minority of *Ixodes scapularis* (or on the west coast, *Ixodes pacificus*) ticks are infected with *Borrelia burgdorferi* (see Chapter 1, "Epidemiology, Ecology, and Prevention of Lyme Disease"). In general, only the nymphal- and adult-stage ticks are capable of transmitting disease. Unfed larvae are very rarely infected with *B. burgdorferi;* ticks can only become infected from a host in the environment; infection cannot be transmitted vertically from a tick to its offspring.

The duration of tick attachment is another factor in transmission of infection. In most circumstances, simple removal of a tick will prevent transmission, even if the tick is infected (2). In mice, a tick attached for less than

48 hours is unlikely to transmit *B. burgdorferi* (3). This delay in transmission probably results from the fact that the tick must ingest a blood meal before infection can be transmitted. Unfed ticks harbor *B. burgdorferi* in their midgut, whereas transmission of infection occurs from the tick salivary gland (4). After the tick has ingested a blood meal, the spirochetes in the midgut are activated to replicate and cause systemic infection in the tick. The salivary gland of the tick becomes infected, thus enabling the tick to become a competent vector that can transmit infecting organisms to the host.

Development of Erythema Migrans

Ticks attach to hosts through a process called questing. They generally are found in grasses, often at the edge of wooded areas. They neither jump nor fly, so initial contact is generally around the ankle level. They may attach at the initial point of contact or move about until they encounter an obstruction before attempting to attach. Groin, popliteal fossae, gluteal folds, axillary folds, and ear lobe creases (especially in children) are common sites of attachment. The tick bite may go unnoticed, as has been the case for most persons enrolled in Lyme disease treatment studies historically. It also appears that some persons do not develop localized infection but instead have systemic inoculation directly into the bloodstream at disease onset.

If *B. burgdorferi* is transmitted through a tick bite ("bite" is actually a misnomer since the tick must be attached and feeding for hours to days), then the initial site of infection in the new host is the skin at the site of the bite. After a period of incubation varying from a few days to as long as a few weeks, the slowly replicating spirochetes cause a gradually spreading localized infection in skin characterized by an expanding annular skin lesion. Lesions are warm to the touch, generally sharply demarcated, blanch on pressure, and are nontender to minimally tender, although many patients describe a tingling or sensitivity (1). Spirochetes can be isolated from skin lesions by culture of skin biopsy samples in appropriate media. Spirochetal DNA has also been demonstrated by polymerase chain reaction (PCR) of processed skin lesion biopsy samples (5).

The average diameter attained by untreated EM lesions is 15 cm, with some achieving diameters of 30 cm or more (1). The rate of expansion is slower than that of cellulitis, generally on the order of 1 to 2 cm per day. Some lesions are atypical in appearance, with central induration, vesiculation, or ulceration or with a variation in color, such as a bluish hue rather than the more typical erythematous appearance.

It is important to recognize that not all tick-transmitted spreading erythemas are caused by *B. burgdorferi* infection. A recent report describes a careful analysis of a series of persons with annular erythemas occurring after tick bites in Missouri (6). The clinical description of their lesions was consistent with EM and therefore met the case definition of Lyme disease. Analysis with serologic testing, culture, and PCR, however, did not show any link with *B. burgdorferi* infection, and the area of exposure has not been documented to be endemic (6). It is very likely that an as-yet-unidentified, tick-transmitted organism rather than Lyme disease is responsible for the illness in these patients. The same may be true of sporadic cases of so-called "Lyme disease" reported from other nonendemic areas. Culture confirmation of cases in areas not previously known to be endemic is therefore very important.

Acute Disseminated Lyme Disease

In addition to causing a spreading localized infection in skin, organisms may seed the bloodstream (not surprisingly, since the ticks are obtaining a blood meal) and cause a variety of systemic symptoms and secondary sites of infection. Among persons infected with *B. burgdorferi* who do not receive antibiotic treatment, 20% develop only erythema migrans without later manifestations of disease (7). The cardinal signs of dissemination are systemic toxicity (fever, chills, arthralgia, myalgia, headache) and the development of secondary skin lesions. Secondary lesions occurred in 50% of persons with *B. burgdorferi* infection in the original natural history studies of Lyme disease conducted at Yale (8). These lesions resemble primary lesions but may occur anywhere on the body and generally expand less than primary lesions. *B. burgdorferi* has been cultured from secondary lesions. The constellation of systemic symptoms has been described as flu-like, a term that has been misleading for some because of the absence in Lyme disease of clinically significant pharyngitis or cough and the usual absence of gastrointestinal symptoms (Case 2.1).

The symptoms accompanying disease dissemination indicate ongoing infection and the immune response engendered by the infecting organism. This phase of illness spontaneously remits after usually no longer than 1 month in untreated persons. Sometimes, however, major organs become involved before remission. Skin lesions do resolve without treatment, as do fever and generalized symptoms such as arthralgia and myalgia. The ten-

---

CASE 2.1 *Flu-like illness with erythema migrans*

A 27- year-old man presents with headache and generalized achiness 1 week after returning from a camping trip in southern New England. On physical examination, his temperature is 101 °F (38 °C) and an erythematous annular patch 8 cm in diameter is present in the right popliteal fossa.

dency to disseminate seems to be greater with some species of *B. burgdorferi* than with others. As with other infectious diseases, both host factors and the characteristics of the particular infecting organism affect the course of the disease.

Another emerging tick-transmitted disease that may be confused with disseminated Lyme disease is human ehrlichiosis. Most cases of ehrlichiosis occur in the southcentral or southeastern United States and are associated with *Amblyomma americanum* or *Dermacentor variabilis* tick bites. Typical symptoms of ehrlichiosis include fever, chills, headache, nausea, myalgia, arthralgia, fatigue, and rash. Rashes are pleomorphic and may be petechial, macular, or papular; some patients have diffuse erythema without distinct rash. Leukopenia and thrombocytopenia are common, as are abnormalities in liver function tests. Diagnosis can be confirmed by an increase in antibody titers in specific serologic testing. The infection responds promptly to treatment with tetracycline (9,10). It is easy to see how ehrlichiosis and disseminated Lyme disease may be confused.

In untreated cases, Lyme disease disseminates to major organs shortly after disease onset, even though that dissemination may remain clinically silent for months or even years. Organ systems affected preferentially are the nervous system, heart, and joints. Much less commonly, eye structures (11,12), the liver (13), skeletal muscle (14), subcutaneous tissues (15), and the spleen (16) have been sites of infection.

Neurologic Manifestations

B. burgdorferi infection can affect multiple neurologic structures, including the meninges, brain, spinal cord, spinal and peripheral nerves, and nerve roots (17,18). Studies using PCR and culture have demonstrated that the central nervous system can be seeded early in the course of disease, with such infection being heralded by relatively minor symptoms such as headache and transient paresthesias (19,20). The most common acute neurologic abnormalities are facial nerve palsy, meningitis, and radiculoneuropathy which, alone or in combination, occur in 15% of untreated patients (18). Acute neurologic abnormalities generally appear within the first few weeks to months after onset of infection. Other cranial nerve palsies also occur but are much less common than facial nerve paralysis. The prognosis of these acute abnormalities is excellent. In the pre-antibiotic era of Lyme disease, they all were shown to remit spontaneously, with complete recovery being the rule. Facial nerve paralysis resolves completely in more than 90% of patients (21). Meningitis also remits, although it often waxes and wanes for weeks to months before resolving completely. In a group of patients followed prospectively, radiculoneuropathy resolved with anti-inflammatory treatment alone over a period of 3 to 18 months (18).

Polymerase chain reaction and culture data indicate that neurologic abnormalities are associated with central nervous system infection in a significant number of persons—probably all persons with meningitis and most with radiculoneuropathy and cranial neuropathy. It is not clear whether central nervous system infection accompanies all cases of peripheral or cranial neuropathy (22). Natural history data are not available to determine whether spontaneous remission of symptoms and signs is associated with resolution of infection or whether infection persists in a latent fashion unless antibiotic therapy is administered.

Cardiac Manifestations

Lyme carditis generally occurs during the same phase of illness as acute neurologic abnormalities (23). A small number of persons with carditis have been studied with endomyocardial biopsy (24) and electrodiagnostic studies (25). In these patients, the biopsies were interpreted as demonstrating direct myocardial invasion, and the electrophysiologic data indicated widespread involvement of the conduction system.

Clinical manifestations classically involve the conduction system, with the sudden occurrence of high-grade atrioventricular block resulting in palpitations, light headedness, and syncope. Most patients with Lyme carditis in recent years have presented with cardiac manifestations only, EM either not occurring or being missed (26). Mobitz type 1 atrioventricular block (AV Wenckebach) has been most common.

Dilated cardiomyopathy or reversible ventricular impairment that is attributed to diffuse myocardial involvement (27) has been described, but in general, Lyme carditis causes conduction system abnormalities without generalized impairment of contractility. No valvular lesions have been described, nor has symptomatic pericarditis. The absence of valvular lesions makes it possible to distinguish Lyme carditis from acute rheumatic fever and bacterial endocarditis.

Early observational studies demonstrated that carditis occurred in 5% to 10% of patients with untreated Lyme disease (with EM as the marker of disease onset) and that cardiac abnormalities resolved with antibiotic therapy, observation, aspirin, or glucocorticoids. No long-term cardiac sequelae have been attributed to cardiac involvement in Lyme disease.

Arthritis

Acute arthritis also may begin during the phase of acute disseminated Lyme disease. The first attacks of acute inflammatory arthritis may occur as early as a few weeks to a few months after disease onset (8). Classically, however, arthritis has been considered a sign of late-stage disease. The typical acute arthritis attack is monoarticular with only one knee being affected in 80% of patients. Sudden pain and swelling with massive effusions, up to 100 mL or more, are common (Case 2.2). The attack begins suddenly and remits after a few days to a few weeks in most patients (median, 8 days) even without antibiotic therapy. Most patients experience recurrent attacks in the same joint, with three or fewer joints affected overall. Although some patients have continuous joint inflammation from the outset, most experience intermittent attacks (7). This pattern of intermittent acute inflammatory arthritis suggests an immunologic process.

Culture (28), histologic staining (29), and PCR data (30) all indicate that, before the patient receives therapy, involved joints are infected with *B. burgdorferi*. Over time, inflammation becomes chronic in a minority of patients. HLA-DR4 may identify those persons at particular risk for developing chronic arthritis after an initial attack of Lyme arthritis (31). The development of chronic arthritis has been shown to be associated with an immune response against a certain outer-surface protein of *B. burgdorferi* (outer-surface protein A) (32). The implications of this finding are uncertain at present but suggest an interplay between local infection and immunologic response in persons in whom continuing inflammation develops.

Taken together, the best hypothesis at present suggests that the infection begins in the skin in most, if not all, patients. Some persons, however, have direct inoculation into the bloodstream rather than localized infection. In a minority of patients, the infection is controlled by the host's immune response, but in most, infection spreads through the bloodstream to a variety of organs, especially the nervous system, heart, and joints. Clinical manifestations evolve over weeks to months or even years in a relatively indolent fashion.

Although the time of dissemination to various organs is not known for certain, it seems most likely that organisms disseminate soon after disease onset and remain clinically silent until some triggering event leads to a strong inflammatory response and clinical manifestations of infection. The inflammatory response is associated with a prominent immunologic component but has little tendency for tissue destruction. In any individual or-

---

CASE 2.2 *Monoarticular inflammatory arthritis with massive effusion*

A 43-year-old man abruptly develops painful swelling of his right knee during mid-November after doing yard work over the weekend at his home in Long Island. He has no history of knee injury. On physical examination, he is found to have a large effusion that limits full flexion, and the right knee is warm to the touch. Joint aspiration yields 50 mL of yellow cloudy fluid with 20,000 leukocytes/mL and 1000 erythrocytes/mL.

gan, inflammation tends to remit without antibiotic therapy, possibly in response to control or containment of local infection, but without eradication of the infection. Inflammation during acute disseminated Lyme disease therefore tends to be intermittent and nonprogressive.

Chronic (Late) Lyme Disease

Over time, the pattern of episodic inflammation may be replaced by a more indolent, persistent inflammation in the nervous system or joints. The term chronic, or late, Lyme disease is generally used to describe continuous inflammation in a specific organ system for more than 1 year. Chronic inflammation also may occur in skin, causing acrodermatitis chronica atrophicans, an atrophic, violaceous lesion usually found on distal extremities at the site of a tick bite. Acrodermatitis chronica atrophicans is caused more commonly by some species of *B. burgdorferi* than others and is more common in Europe than in the United States (33).

The diagnosis of late Lyme disease is often made after a prolonged period of latency or minimally symptomatic disease. When questioned closely, most patients with late neurologic disease describe having had low-grade, continuing symptoms for several months before diagnosis (headache, sleep disturbance, subtle difficulty concentrating, energy depletion, tingling in extremities) rather than true disease latency. The full spectrum of chronic or late Lyme disease is a matter of current debate and active study.

Chronic Arthritis

Chronic Lyme arthritis is characterized by persistent inflammatory arthritis of one to a few joints, most often the knee. The risk of developing chronic arthritis appears to be greater in persons who are HLA-DR4 positive (31). The shift from episodic arthritis to chronic arthritis in this group is associated with the development of an immune response to one of the outer-surface proteins (OspA) of the spirochete. Inflammation in chronically affected joints often does not subside after antibiotic therapy, and study with PCR has not revealed gene sequences of *B. burgdorferi* in the joint fluid of persons with persistent arthritis after treatment with prolonged courses of oral or intravenous antibiotics (*see* Chapter 6) (30). These observations suggest that chronic Lyme arthritis may not be due to persistent infection.

The histologic lesion of chronic Lyme arthritis mimics that of rheumatoid arthritis. Synovial tissue samples reveal synovial hypertrophy, neovascularity, infiltration by macrophages, and a mixed population of lymphocytes with a perivascular distribution. Even chronic inflammation may resolve spontaneously occasionally after many years of persistent arthritis.

Chronic (Late) Neurologic Disease

Chronic neurologic Lyme disease (sometimes called tertiary neuroborreliosis) has been particularly difficult to study because of the prolonged time course over which it evolves and the subtle nature of the clinical manifestations in most persons. The two best described manifestations are a subtle sensoriradiculoneuropathy and a low-grade encephalopathy (34). Nerve biopsies in persons with neuropathy have shown perineural inflammation in a pattern that is not unique to Lyme disease. Whether *B. burgdorferi* directly invades peripheral nerves is unclear at present. The neuropathy is usually not progressive and responds inconsistently to antibiotic therapy. The diagnosis is based on laboratory confirmation of Lyme disease and the elimination of other potential causes.

The symptoms that can be attributed to encephalopathy are limited to cognitive function, with most patients reporting deficits in ability to concentrate, learning, and short-term memory (Case 2.3) (34,35). Cerebrospinal fluid samples generally show some degree of inflammatory response, with elevation in total protein or low-grade pleocytosis.

Chronic neurologic lesions can be linked to Lyme disease only through direct detection of the organism in the central nervous system or through indirect means (measurement of a specific immunologic response in serum or spinal fluid). Antigen capture assays and PCR have been used to help diagnose neurologic Lyme disease. In routine clinical settings, however, laboratory confirmation is based on serologic testing combined with confirmatory Western immunoblotting and measurement of antibody levels in cerebrospinal fluid (36).

A range of other neurologic lesions have been attributed to *B. burgdorferi* infection, although much less commonly. These include encephalomyelopathy, focal encephalitis, and optic neuritis, with case reports linking other lesions based on immunoreactivity to *B. burgdorferi*.

CASE 2.3 *Chronic peripheral neuropathy with mild encephalopathy*

A 53-year-old woman presents with a history of several months of difficulty sleeping, difficulty concentrating, and fatigue. She also has symptoms of tingling in distal aspects of both lower extremities. The results of the physical examination are normal except for a slight decrease in pin prick in a stocking distribution bilaterally. The results of the mental status examination are within normal limits. Formal psychometric testing, however, reveals a selective deficit in short-term memory. Electromyography shows mildly abnormal results with normal nerve conduction studies.

Differential Diagnosis

There has been much debate regarding the relationship between chronic fatigue syndrome, fibromyalgia, and Lyme disease. Small series have demonstrated that fibromyalgia may occur as a sequela to Lyme disease and that Lyme disease may trigger that disorder (37,38). The exact relationship remains speculative, however, and is complicated by the fact that fibromyalgia is such an extraordinarily common disorder in general practice. The clinical characteristics of chronic Lyme disease and fibromyalgia are contrasted in Table 2.1. Fibromyalgia may complicate any chronic pain state. It should be recognized as a distinct entity that is not necessarily related to Lyme disease in any specific fashion.

Prognosis

Population-based studies to evaluate the general health status of persons with previous Lyme disease have suggested that a history of Lyme disease is associated with lower long-term general health status compared with that

Table 2.1   Comparison of Chronic Lyme Disease and Fibromyalgia

Characteristic	Chronic Lyme Disease	Fibromyalgia
Neurologic	Cognitive impairment	Fatigue
	Short-term memory deficit	Nonrestorative sleep
	Distal paresthesias	Frequent nocturnal awakenings
	Fatigue	
Musculoskeletal	Arthralgia and inflammatory monoarticular or oligoarticular, large-joint arthritis	Widespread pain in axial distribution
	Predilection for knee(s)	Bilateral distribution, both above and below the waist
		Tender points at characteristic periarticular sites
Serologic	IgG antibodies against B. burgdorferi	No relationship to seroreactivity against B. burgdorferi
Responsiveness to antibiotic therapy	Gradual improvement or arresting of progression after 4-week course	Unresponsive to antibiotic therapy

of matched controls (39). Much further study is needed to determine whether the differences in general health status reflect continued infection, post-infectious sequelae, or fixed deficits resulting from previous infection.

Summary

Lyme disease is an emerging illness with manifestations that commonly span months and even years. Because the disease has been recognized only relatively recently and because of its prolonged clinical course, new late disease manifestations may become apparent in the future. To date, most of our understanding can be attributed to clinical observation, epidemiologic study, and treatment trials, investigative methods that cannot shed light on basic disease mechanisms.

Many questions remain. How does the organism evade immunologic destruction? What is occurring during periods of apparent disease latency? What is the mechanism of chronic neurologic and joint disease? What is the full spectrum of late disease manifestations, and what is the optimal treatment of these manifestations? Does the illness ever become self-perpetuating? Does spontaneous resolution of clinical manifestations reflect cure or latency? What characteristics of the organism and host determine the course of the illness?

It is hoped that investigations in progress will provide answers to these and other questions about Lyme disease. What is learned through the study of Lyme disease holds promise to shed light on other idiopathic chronic neurologic and joint diseases.

■   ■   ■

Key Points

- Lyme disease is a vector-borne disease caused by *Borrelia burgdorferi* and transmitted to humans by ixodid ticks.
- Disease onset is heralded by appearance of a characteristic skin lesion, erythema migrans, at the site of a tick bite.
- Disease course is highly variable and evolves gradually over weeks (acute disseminated disease) to months (acute neurologic manifestations, acute arthritis and carditis) and even years (chronic arthritis and neurologic manifestations).
- Diagnosis is based on clinical features supported by confirmatory serologic data.

■   ■   ■

REFERENCES

1. **Steere AC, Bartenhagen NH, Craft JE, et al.** The early clinical manifestations of Lyme disease. Ann Intern Med. 1983;99:76-82.

2. **Shapiro ED, Gerber MA, Holabird NB, et al.** A controlled trial of antimicrobial prophylaxis for Lyme disease after deer-tick bites. N Engl J Med. 1992;327:1769-73.

3. **Piesman J, Mather TN, Sinsky RJ, Spielman A.** Duration of tick attachment and *Borrelia burgdorferi* transmission. J Clin Microbiol. 1987;25:557-8.

4. **Piesman J.** Dispersal of the Lyme disease spirochete *Borrelia burgdorferi* to salivary glands of feeding nymphal *Ixodes scapularis* (Acari: Ixodidae). J Med Entomol. 1995;32:5l9-21.

5. **Schwartz I, Wormser GP, Schwartz JJ, et al.** Diagnosis of early Lyme disease by polymerase chain reaction application and culture of skin biopsies from erythema migrans lesions. J Clin Microbiol. 1992;30:3082-8.

6. **Campbell GL, Paul WS, Schriefer ME, et al.** Epidemiologic and diagnostic studies of patients with suspected early Lyme disease, Missouri, 1990–1993. J Infect Dis. 1995;172:470-80.

7. **Steere AC, Schoen RT, Taylor E.** The clinical evolution of Lyme arthritis. Ann Intern Med. 1987;107:725-31.

8. **Steere AC, Malawista SE, Hardin JA, et al.** Erythema chronicum migrans and Lyme arthritis. Ann Intern Med. 1977;86:685-98.

9. **Everett ED, Evans KA, Henry RB, McDonald G.** Human ehrlichiosis in adults after tick exposure. Ann Intern Med. 1994;120:730-5.

10. **Fishbein DB, Dawson JE, Robinson LE.** Human ehrlichiosis in the United States, 1985 to 1990. Ann Intern Med. 1994;120:726-43.

11. **Aaberg TM.** The expanding ophthalmologic spectrum of Lyme disease. Am J Ophthalmol. 1989;107:77-80.

12. **Lesser RL, Kornmehl EW, Pachner AR, et al.** Neuro-ophthalmologic manifestations of Lyme disease. Ophthalmology 1990;97:699-706.

13. **Goellner MH, Agger WA, Burgess JH, Duray PH.** Hepatitis due to recurrent Lyme disease. Ann Intern Med. 1988;108:707-8.

14. **Atlas E, Novak SN, Duray PH, Steere AC.** Lyme myositis: muscle invasion by *Borrelia burgdorferi*. Ann Intern Med. 1988;109:245-6.

15. **Kramer N, Rickert RR, Brodkin RH, Rosenstein ED.** Septal panniculitis as a manifestation of Lyme disease. Am J Med. 1986;81:149-52.

16. **Rank EL, Dias SM, Hasson J, et al.** Human necrotizing splenitis caused by *Borrelia burgdorferi*. Am J Clin Pathol. 1989;91:493-8.

17. **Reik L, Steere AC, Bartenhagen NH, et al.** Neurologic abnormalities of Lyme disease. Medicine. 1979;58:281-94.

18. **Pachner AR, Steere AC.** The triad of neurologic manifestations of Lyme disease: meningitis, cranial neuritis, and radiculoneuritis. Neurology. 1985;35:47-53.

19. **Luft BJ, Steinman CR, Neimark HC, et al.** Invasion of the central nervous system by *Borrelia burgdorferi* in acute disseminated infection. JAMA. 1992;267:1364-7.

20. **Pfister HW, Preac-Mursic V, Wilske B, et al.** Latent Lyme neuroborreliosis: presence of *Borrelia burgdorferi* in the cerebrospinal fluid without concurrent inflammatory signs. Neurology. 1989;39:1118-20.

21. **Clark JR, Carlson RD, Packner AR, et al.** Facial paralysis in Lyme disease. Laryngoscope 1985;95:1341-5.

22. **Keller TL, Halperin JJ, Whitman M.** PCR detection of *Borrelia burgdorferi* DNA in cerebrospinal fluid of Lyme neuroborreliosis patients. Neurology 1992;42:32-42.

23. **Steere AC, Batsford WP, Weinberg M, et al.** Lyme carditis: cardiac abnormalities of Lyme disease. Ann Intern Med. 1980;93:8-16.

24. **de koning J, Hoogkamp-Korstanje JAA, van der Linde MR, Crijns HJGM.** Demonstration of spirochetes in cardiac biopsies of patients with Lyme disease. J Infect Dis. 1989;160:150-2.

25. **van der Linde MR, Crijns HJGM, de Koning J, et al.** Range of atrioventricular conduction disturbances in Lyme borreliosis: a report of four cases and review of other published reports. Br Heart J 1990;63:162-8.

26. **McAlister HF, Klementowicz PT, Andrews C, et al.** Lyme carditis: an important cause of reversible heart block. Ann Intern Med 1989;110:339-45.

27. **Stanek G, Klein J, Bittner R, Glogar D.** Isolation of *Borrelia burgdorferi* from the myocardium of a patient with long-standing cardiomyopathy. N Engl J Med. 1990;322:249-52.

28. **Snydman DR, Schenkein DP, Berardi VP, et al.** *Borrelia burgdorferi* in joint fluid in chronic Lyme arthritis. Ann Intern Med. 1986;104:798-800.

29. **Johnson JE, Duray PH, Steere AC, et al.** Lyme arthritis: spirochetes found in synovial microangiopathic lesions. Am J Pathol. 1985;118:26-34.

30. **Nocton JJ, Dressler F, Rutledge BJ, et al.** Detection of *Borrelia burgdorferi* DNA by polymerase chain reaction in synovial fluid from patients with Lyme arthritis. N Engl J Med 1994;330:229-34.

31. **Steere AC, Dwyer E, Winchester R.** Association of chronic Lyme arthritis with HLA-DR4 and HLA-DR2 alleles. N Engl J Med. 1990;323:219-23.

32. **Kalish RA, Leong JM, Steere AC.** Association of treatment-resistant chronic Lyme arthritis with HLA-DR4 and antibody reactivity to OspA and OspB of *Borrelia burgdorferi.* Infect Immun 1993;61:2774-9.

33. **Kaufman LD, Gruber BL, Phillips ME, Benach JL.** Late cutaneous Lyme disease: acrodermatitis chronica atrophicans. Am J Med. 1989;86:828-30.

34. **Logigian EL, Kaplan RF, Steere AC.** Chronic neurologic manifestation of Lyme disease. N Engl J Med. 1990;323:1438-4.

35. **Halperin JJ, Luft BJ, Anand AK, et al.** Lyme neuroborreliosis: central nervous system manifestations. Neurology 1989;39:753-9.

36. **Steere AC, Berardi VP, Weeks KE, et al.** Evaluation of the intrathecal antibody response to *Borrelia burgdorferi* as a diagnostic test for Lyme neuroborreliosis. J Infect Dis. 1990;161:12039.

37. **Dinerman H, Steere AC.** Lyme disease associated with fibromyalgia. Ann Intern Med. 1992;117:281-5.

38. **Hsu VM, Patella SJ, Sigal LH.** Chronic Lyme disease as the incorrect diagnosis in patients with fibromyalgia. Arthritis Rheum. 1993;36:493-1500.

39. **Shadick NA, Phillips CB, Logigian EL, et al.** The long-term clinical outcomes of Lyme disease. Ann Intern Med. 1994;121:560-7.

KEY REFERENCES

Pachner AR, Steere AC. The triad of neurologic manifestations of Lyme disease: meningitis, cranial neuritis, and radiculoneuritis. Neurology. 1985;35:47-53.

This paper characterizes the acute neurologic manifestations of Lyme disease in North America. The unique features of inflammation of central nervous system meninges and peripheral nerves are described.

Steere AC, Bartenhagen NH, Craft JE, et al. The early clinical manifestations of Lyme disease. Ann Intern Med. 1983;99:76-82.

The most complete description of early Lyme disease. The complete range of symptoms associated with erythema migrans is described.

Steere AC, Grodzicki RL, Kornblatt AN, et al. The spirochetal etiology of Lyme disease. N Engl J Med. 1983;99:76-82.

This landmark paper describes the definitive identification of Borrelia burgdorferi *as the cause of Lyme disease. The growth of the causative agent on the culture and the development of a serologic test to confirm the diagnosis are over-reported.*

Steere AC, Malawista SE, Syndman DR, et al. Lyme arthritis: an epidemic of oligoarticular arthritis in children and adults in three Connecticut communities. Arthritis. Rheum. 1977;20:7-17.

The first description of an epidemic of inflammatory arthritis in regions around Lyme, Connecticut.

Steere AC, Schoen RT, Taylor E. The clinical evolution of Lyme arthritis. Ann Intern Med. 1987;107:725-31.

The natural history and clinical spectrum of Lyme arthritis are reported in this classic report. The evolution from arthralgias, through acute, intermittent, inflammatory arthritis of the knees, to chronic persistent arthritis in a minority of persons is described.

3

■ ■ ■

Management of Tick
Bites and Early Lyme Disease

Robert B. Nadelman, MD

Gary P. Wormser, MD

Early recognition of the bite of an *Ixodes scapularis* (formerly *Ixodes dammini*) tick and rapid removal of an attached tick may prevent Lyme disease. The risk of infection after a tick bite, however, is small (<5%), and routine prophylactic therapy is not currently recommended. If an erythema migrans rash appears, treatment with oral antibiotics such as doxycycline or amoxicillin is effective in resolving symptoms and preventing extracutaneous complications.

Management of Tick Bites

Tick Removal and Immediate Management

Early recognition of an *I. scapularis* (formerly *I. dammini*) tick bite and rapid removal of an attached tick may prevent Lyme disease. Attached ticks do not disengage when subjected to water pressure in the shower and may be difficult to remove by hand. Attempting to force out the tick with a flame, fingernail polish, 70% isopropyl alcohol, or petroleum jelly is also ineffective (1) and may result in injury. A fine-toothed "jeweler's" forceps is an effective means of removing attached ticks. Forceps should be disinfected before and after use and should not be shared. The steps in using the forceps for tick removal are as follows:

1.   Insert the forceps tip at the point where the tick mouth parts are attached to the skin.

2.   Apply steady upward pressure (without twisting [1]) to dis-
lodge the tick (2,3). Avoid squeezing the tick's body, to prevent forcing its contents into the host (1).

3.   After the tick has been dislodged, remove any remaining
mouth parts separately; this can usually be done with minimal
trauma to the skin. A small shave excision has sometimes been
recommended for residual tick parts, but this procedure is
probably not necessary (2).

4.   Clean the area of the bite with soap and water. The use of topical
antibiotics for patients in whom tick mouth parts remain embed-
ded (2) has not been formally studied but may be considered.

Assessing the Risk of Lyme Disease After a Tick Bite

To develop a sensible approach to managing the patient with an *I. scapularis* tick bite (but *without* evidence of illness), the clinician must first be
able to recognize this tick and understand the likelihood of illness caused
by its bite.

Identification of *I. scapularis* ticks is reviewed in Chapter 1, "Epidemiology, Ecology, and Prevention of Lyme Disease." Patients reporting tick
bites should be asked to save the tick (ideally in a jar filled with alcohol)
and bring it for identification. Many "ticks" are actually spiders, scabs, or
dirt, and thus pose no risk of Lyme disease (4,5). Ticks other than *I. scapularis*, including *Dermacentor variabilis* (dog tick) and *Amblyomma americanum* (lone star tick), do not transmit *Borrelia burgdorferi* and thus pose
little or no risk of Lyme disease (6) (although such ticks may carry other
pathogens [6–8]).

Lyme disease is most often transmitted by the bite of nymphal-stage *I.
scapularis* ticks. However, the overwhelming majority of such bites (probably >95%) do *not* result in transmission of Lyme disease (9–14). Because
this rate of transmission is considerably less than the rate of *B. burgdorferi*
infection in nymphal ticks (25% to 30% in some endemic areas) (2,15), factors other than the bite of infected tick itself must be important in contracting infection (Table 3.1). Also, although adult *I. scapularis* are twice as
likely as nymphal *I. scapularis* ticks to be infected with *B. burgdorferi*,
adult ticks play a much smaller role in transmission of Lyme disease to humans (2,15) (see Chapter 1, "Epidemiology, Ecology, and Prevention of
Lyme Disease").

The relatively small likelihood of acquiring Lyme disease from *I. pacificus*, the principal vector on the west coast of the United States, is partly
due to the low infection rate in this tick species (16). Lyme disease is also
unlikely to occur after the bite of larval-stage *I. scapularis* ticks, because *I.
scapularis* ticks at this stage do not carry *B. burgdorferi* (17).

Table 3.1   Factors Influencing the Risk of Contracting Lyme Disease in the United States

Risk Factor	High Risk
Geography	Endemic area for both vector tick and *B. burgdorferi*
Season	Late spring, summer (for Northeast and Midwest) (U.S.)
Tick species	*Ixodes scapularis*
	Ixodes pacificus (West Coast) (U.S.)
Tick stage	Nymph
Duration of tick feeding	≥48 h (tick feeds to partial engorgement)
Strain variation in *B. burgdorferi*	Presence of putative virulence factors*
Host immunity (native or vaccine induced)	Absence of host immunity*
Host anti-tick antibody	Absence of host anti-tick antibody*

*The importance of these factors in influencing risk of Lyme disease has not been established in humans.

Factors Influencing the Acquisition of Infection

The role of host immune function on the development of infection is still not well understood. We are investigating whether HLA haplotype influences the clinical outcome in untreated patients who have been bitten by *Ixodes* ticks. Another group has studied the role of humoral immunity to the tick itself in high-risk outdoor workers (18). They have postulated that human antibody-associated hypersensitivity reactions to proteins in tick saliva might induce pruritus, prompting a person to detect and remove a tick before infection occurs (18).

Other considerations include biologic factors related to the spirochete itself. One recent investigation has suggested that spirochete transmission from tick vectors may depend on virulence factors that are present only in certain strains of *B. burgdorferi* (19).

The most compelling evidence to date, however, suggests that duration of tick feeding is the crucial determinant of transmission. Unlike the rapid transmission (<1 hour) of *Borrelia* species by the soft tick vectors of relapsing fever (20), transmission of *B. burgdorferi* by *I. scapularis* (hard ticks) probably takes days. In experimental animal systems (21) and humans (5), *I. scapularis* rarely transmitted infection before 48 hours of attachment. This long period may partly reflect the time required for putative host factors ingested during the blood meal to activate virulence factors in *B. burgdorferi* (22), the time needed for multiplication of *B. burgdorferi* to a minimal infectious inoculum, and/or the time required for spirochetes to pass from the tick midgut to salivary glands (22) (*see* Chapter 9, "Lyme Disease Vaccine"). Spirochete transmission may occur more rapidly if *partially fed* ticks are allowed to reattach to feed on new hosts (23). However, the relevance of this finding to the clinical setting is uncertain.

Nevertheless, from a practical clinical standpoint, it is difficult to determine the duration of tick attachment. Patient estimates are often unreliable (5,24). More reliable is a measurement of tick engorgement (scutal index) (5,25), but this technique requires considerable expertise.

Testing for Spirochetes in Ticks

Detection of spirochetes in a tick by polymerase chain reaction (PCR) or other methods has not yet been shown to provide clinically useful information. Since transmission of infection probably takes more than 48 hours, detection of spirochetes in the tick does not necessarily indicate that human infection has occurred. The absence of detectable spirochetes in a tick does not signify that infection cannot occur, because blood inhibitors may interfere with PCR (5,26) or spirochetes may already have been transmitted.

PCR assays also have not been standardized and may yield false-positive results because of contamination. At present, the role of examining ticks for spirochetes should be confined to research studies rather than serve as a guide to management of individual patients with tick bites.

Antibiotic Prophylaxis After Tick Bites

The value of antibiotic prophylaxis depends on its efficacy in preventing Lyme disease versus the risks and economic costs associated with the use of these drugs. Even if antibiotics were not associated with any adverse consequences, were 100% effective in preventing Lyme disease after a tick bite, and were uniformly administered to everyone who reported an *I. scapularis* bite, less than one-third of Lyme disease cases would be averted. This is because only 14% to 32% of North American patients actually recall receiving an *I. scapularis* bite (27–30).

Ixodes scapularis bites often go unnoticed for several reasons. Nymphal-stage *I. scapularis* ticks may easily be overlooked because of their small size and the absence of significant tenderness or pruritus associated with their bite. In addition, the bites most likely to result in Lyme disease occur on those parts of the body where a tick can feed unnoticed for several days. These areas include such difficult to visualize sites as the popliteal fossae, buttocks, axillae, groin, and back.

Although a number of antibiotics are effective in treating Lyme disease, no study to date has demonstrated that antibiotic prophylaxis reduces the risk of Lyme disease when given to patients after an *Ixodes* bite, possibly because of insufficient enrollment of volunteers (i.e., type II error). Even a meta-analysis of three randomized placebo-controlled studies involving 600 participants (10–12) failed to demonstrate efficacy of antibiotic prophylaxis (pooled odds ratio 0.0; $P = 0.12$ [95% CI, 0.0 to 1.5]) (31).

The risk of adverse effects from antibiotics must be considered in any decision to use these drugs in tick bite management. *The risk of acquiring Lyme disease after a tick bite has been observed to be equal to the risk of developing adverse effects caused by the prophylactic antibiotics* (10,11). Photosensitivity caused by doxycycline may exceed 15% during the summer months (32). The possibility of drug-drug interactions, *Clostridium difficile*–associated diarrhea, superinfections (e.g., *Candida* vaginitis), antimicrobial resistance, cost factors, and patient inconvenience must also be considered, especially because many residents of endemic areas are bitten repeatedly during the summer months (13) and thus would be taking antibiotics for weeks or even for months. For instance, it has been estimated that more than 150,000 *I. scapularis* bites occur annually in Westchester County, New York, alone (33). The use of prophylactic *topical* antibiotics might avoid some of the problems associated with systemic agents, but this has not been formally studied in humans (34).

Concerns have been raised that untreated tick bites will ultimately lead to significant clinical sequelae such as cardiac, rheumatologic, or neurologic disease (14). However, most patients with late-stage Lyme disease are believed to have had antecedent erythema migrans (EM), a readily identifiable lesion, at the site of the bite (14,35–38). Among more than 1,000 participants followed in prospective studies at our center (unpublished data) and elsewhere (10–13), none has been reported to have developed late or latent infection (latent infection is defined as asymptomatic seroconversion, the clinical significance of which is unknown).

Physicians and health care authorities should alert persons with a recognized tick bite to seek medical attention in the event of a **rash** *at the bite site or the onset of slightly less* **fever** *with or without other systemic symptoms such as headache and myalgia. Treatment of EM is highly effective in resolving symptoms and preventing extracutaneous complications of Lyme disease.*

Based on these considerations, the use of prophylactic antibiotics for asymptomatic persons after tick bite is controversial (Table 3.2). Some have proposed prophylactic treatment selectively, including such options as:

1. Treating anxious patients or those unlikely to return for follow-up (39)
2. Treating all persons who remove attached ticks

3. Treating only those with tick bites believed to be high risk (e.g., bites from engorged *I. scapularis* nymphs)

4. Treating only persons who have EM or an illness compatible with Lyme disease

5. Performing serologic tests and treating those whose test results indicate seroconversion

6. Treating selectively high-risk patients, such as pregnant women

A cost-effectiveness analysis, based on a mathematical model, concluded that a 2-week course of doxycycline is indicated for all persons who have removed an attached tick when the probability of *B. burgdorferi* infection after a tick bite is 0.036 or more, and should be an option when the probability ranges from 0.01 to 0.035 (14). However, this particular antibiotic regimen has never been studied clinically in this setting. The authors of several prospective randomized double-blinded clinical studies, in which 600 participants were evaluated, have concluded that *routine antibiotic prophylaxis is not warranted* (10–12). Until more data are available, this remains our approach for most patients.

Because of concerns, however, about fetal wastage and malformations associated with *B. burgdorferi* infection acquired during *pregnancy* (40–42), it is our practice to offer a 10-day course of oral amoxicillin to an asymptomatic pregnant woman who has removed an attached nymphal- or adult-stage *I. scapularis* tick. Even in this specific setting, however, there is no evidence at present that this approach is effective in preventing Lyme disease or that the benefits outweigh the risks (*see* Chapter 7, "Lyme Disease in Children").

Recent evidence suggests that the agent of human granulocytic ehrlichiosis can be transmitted by both the adult and nymphal *I. scapularis* ticks. *Ixodes scapularis* may be co-infected with *B. burgdorferi* and the

Table 3.2   Pros and Cons of the Use of Antimicrobial Therapy for Prevention of Lyme Disease After an *Ixodes scapularis* Tick Bite

Pro	Con
Prevention of illness and extra-cutaneous complications	Efficacy not established
	Risk of adverse effects caused by antibiotics is equal to the risk of Lyme disease after a tick bite
Relief of patient anxiety	
	Cost
	Safety not established

agent of human granulocytic ehrlichiosis (43,44). Further understanding of the transmission and treatment of human granulocytic ehrlichiosis and babesiosis (also transmitted by *I. scapularis*) may modify future recommendations on prophylactic treatment after tick bite.

Erythema Migrans

Clinical Characteristics

Erythema migrans (EM), the rash of early Lyme disease, generally begins as a red macule or papule at the site of the bite of an infected *I. scapularis* tick. The rash expands to form patches of erythema, with or without bands of normal-appearing skin (27,45,46). The initial EM lesion occurs approximately 7 to 10 days (range, 1 to 36 days) after a tick bite, at the site of attachment (27–30). A central papule consisting of several millimeters of erythema, scale, or hyperpigmentation may be observed at the site of the bite (punctum) (Fig. 3.1/Plate 2).

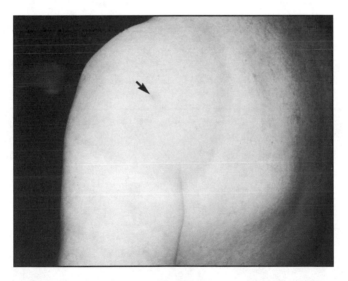

Figure 3.1   Erythema migrans rash with central clearing on the shoulder of a patient. Note central hyperpigmentation at site of tick bite (punctum) (*arrow*). *Borrelia burgdorferi* was isolated from a biopsy culture performed at the periphery of the lesion. (Reprinted with permission from Nadelman RB, Wormser GP. Erythema migrans and early Lyme disease. Am J Med. 1995;98(suppl 4A): 15S–24S.) (For color reproduction, see Plate 2 at back of book.)

The tick has almost always disengaged from the skin by the time the EM rash has developed. For surveillance purposes, the Centers for Disease Control and Prevention (CDC) considers EM lesions to be at least 5 cm in diameter (47). Although this definition is not meant to restrict the diagnosis of an individual patient, it is generally a reliable guide.

A common misconception is that EM must have central clearing. However, of the 59 culture-confirmed EM lesions seen by us for which rash characteristics were recorded, only 37% demonstrated this feature (28) (Fig. 3.2/Plate 3). Central clearing is most commonly seen in patients with long-standing rashes (e.g., rashes of several weeks' duration) (48). The higher frequency of central clearing originally described in the United States may have been related to the longer duration of EM before diagnosis at the time of that report.

EM diameter increases with increased duration of the lesion as the spirochete spreads from the initial tick bite site through the skin (28). Spirochetes are readily isolated from skin biopsy samples taken from the leading margin of EM lesions (28,29,49–51) or from normal-appearing skin adjacent to the lesion (49).

Most EM lesions are oval or round but triangles and other unusual shapes are occasionally seen. The margins are usually regular and generally are not raised compared with the central region. A vesicular center is present in approximately 5% of lesions (Fig. 3.3/Plate 4) (52). Central induration develops in some lesions. Scale is uncommon, occurring primarily in the center at the site of the tick bite, in fading rashes of long duration, or after treatment with antibiotics. The application of topical corticosteroids

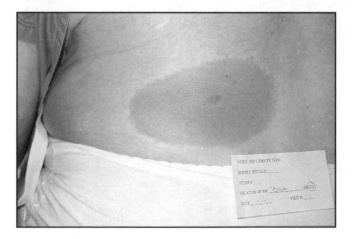

Figure 3.2   Erythema migrans rash without central clearing. *Borrelia burgdorferi* was isolated from a biopsy culture performed at the periphery of the lesion. (For color reproduction, see Plate 3 at back of book.)

may also cause EM lesions to scale or display pallor or both. Lesions in the distal lower extremities may appear purpuric (27).

Hematogenous spread of viable spirochetes may result in one or more secondary lesions (Fig. 3.4/Plate 5). Such lesions may be evanescent, appearing fairly suddenly during an examination and then fading. Prominent local symptoms (pruritus, tenderness, paresthesia), central vesiculation, and postinflammatory changes such as scaling or hyperpigmentation do not occur with secondary lesions.

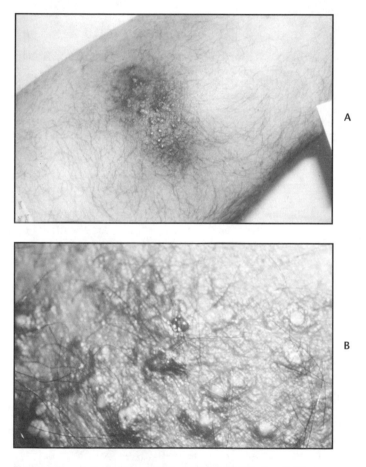

A

B

Figure 3.3   *A*, Vesicular erythema migrans (EM) lesion. *B*, Close-up of same vesicular EM lesion. *Borrelia burgdorferi* was isolated from culture from vesicular fluid (52). (Reprinted with permission from Nadelman RB, Wormser GP. Erythema migrans and early Lyme disease. Am J Med. 1995;98(suppl 4A):15S-24S.) (For color reproduction, see Plate 4 at back of book.)

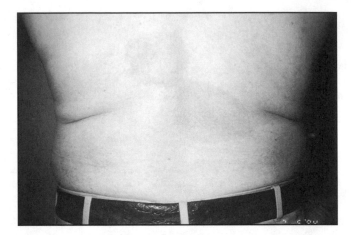

Figure 3.4   Multiple erythema migrans lesions on the back of a patient whose primary lesion is depicted in Figure 3.1. Note the absence of a central papule or postinflammatory skin change. (Reprinted with permission from Nadelman RB, Wormser GP. Erythema migrans and early Lyme disease. Am J Med. 1995;98(suppl 4A):15S-24S.) (For color reproduction, see Plate 5 at back of book.)

Multiple EMs occur in less than 25% of North American patients (27,28,32,53,54). The decreased incidence compared with that originally observed (48%) (30) is probably the result of earlier diagnosis and treatment of Lyme disease in more recent studies.

Associated Symptoms

Most patients with EM (up to 80%) have systemic symptoms; often they are of mild intensity (27,28,30,32,48,53–55). Differences in reported series may be partly related to selection bias. Fatigue (54%), myalgia (44%), arthralgia (44%), headache (42%), fever and/or chills (39%), and stiff neck (35%) were the most common symptoms in a series of 79 culture-confirmed cases (28). The infrequency of respiratory or gastrointestinal symptoms other than anorexia may be an aid to diagnosis.

Symptoms may occur in untreated patients before, concurrent with, or after spontaneous resolution of the rash (27,48,56). Regional lymphadenopathy (23%) and fever (16%) are among the few objective findings besides rash found in patients with EM (28). Cranial nerve palsies and meningitis may occur occasionally with the rash, but objective arthritis typically does not develop in untreated patients until after resolution of EM (mean, 6 mo.) (57).

CASE 3.1   *Erythema migrans unrecognized by a patient with a "viral illness" during the summer*

A 67-year-old man presents in June with symptoms of several days of fever, arthralgia, and profound fatigue. He denies having a cough or gastrointestinal complaints and is unaware of having a rash or previous tick bite. The results of the physical examination are normal except for a temperature of 38 °C and a faint 9 × 9 cm EM lesion on his left buttock. He is prescribed oral doxycycline, 100 mg twice per day for 2 weeks. With this treatment, the patient's symptoms resolve within a few days and do not recur.

Early Lyme Disease Without Erythema Migrans

Widely quoted estimates that EM occurs in 60% to 80% of patients with Lyme disease are based in large part on one study of a small group of patients in an island community (35). *More recent data suggest that EM is recognized in 90% or more of patients with objective Lyme disease* (37,38).

The actual frequency of this rash may be underestimated because of failure to examine the entire skin surface, particularly at body sites that are difficult for patients to visualize. EM may go unnoticed because pruritus, pain, and paresthesia at the site of an EM lesion are usually minimal and thus may not draw attention to the rash.

It is believed that *B. burgdorferi* may occasionally cause a viral-like illness in the absence of EM (58,59), but this has been rare in our experience (see Case 3.1). Persistence of fever and constitutional symptoms that last for more than a few days, absence of respiratory or gastrointestinal complaints, lack of illness in household members, and recent exposure to tick habitats may be clues to the possibility of Lyme disease (58,59), although other tick-borne illnesses such as human granulocytic ehrlichiosis and babesiosis are probably more likely.

Laboratory Diagnosis

Because EM is a clinical diagnosis, serologic testing for antibodies to *B. burgdorferi* is not usually necessary. One half of patients with EM have negative serologic assays at the time of presentation (60). However, approximately 80% of patients with EM who receive treatment will be seropositive at some point during the first month (28,54,61,62). Longer duration of illness is associated with a greater likelihood of initial seropositivity (61,62). In a study of 100 unselected patients seen at our center, of 14 patients with EM of more than 2 weeks' duration, an *initially* positive enzyme-linked immunoassay (ELISA) or immunoblot was present in 13 (93%) and 12 (86%) patients, respectively (62).

Complete blood counts and sedimentation rates are generally normal in patients with Lyme disease. Thrombocytopenia or leukopenia in patients with EM should raise suspicion for co-infection with an additional tick-borne pathogen such as *Babesia microti* or the agent of human granulo-cytic ehrlichiosis (HGE) (63). Liver function assays, however, are mildly abnormal in more than one third of patients with culture-confirmed EM (28). Electrocardiographic evidence of heart block is rare (<5%) (64).

Culture and Polymerase Chain Reaction

Skin-punch biopsies (2 or 4 mm) and aspirates from the leading margin of EM lesions have demonstrated *B. burgdorferi* in up to 88% of patients with clinically diagnosed EM in the United States and Europe (28,29,49,50,65). Excellent culture yields are possible even if specimens are shipped to a separate specialized laboratory for processing, provided that specific trans-port culture medium (modified Barbour-Stoenner-Kelly [BSK]) is used (49,66).

Detection of spirochetes in the blood by culture (58) or by polymerase chain reaction (PCR) (67,68) has a lower yield (usually less than 10% and 30%, respectively). Recent data at our center suggest that if sufficient speci-men volumes are used, blood cultures may be positive in 25% of untreated adult patients with solitary EM lesions (69).

Although PCR has been used to provide microbiologic evidence of in-fection (70), positive PCR signals do not necessarily signify viable organ-isms (see Chapter 10, "Use of the Laboratory in the Confirmation and Management of Lyme Disease"). Strict precautions to avoid laboratory con-tamination are especially important in PCR because of its ability to detect minute amounts of DNA.

Differential Diagnosis

Clues to the diagnosis of EM are outlined in Box 3.1. Erythema migrans must be differentiated from several other disorders (Table 3.3) (46,71). Ery-thema migrans is primarily a disease of the late spring and summer, whereas most other processes occur without seasonal variation.

Localized Tick Bite Reactions

Unlike EM, which usually does not begin for at least several days after a tick has been removed or fallen off (27–30), localized tick bite reactions tend to develop more rapidly. Localized reactions may become quite large within a few hours, greatly exceeding 5 cm, and thus meet the CDC sur-

---

Box 3.1   Clues to the Clinical Diagnosis of Erythema Migrans*†

Epidemiologic

- Travel or residence in an endemic area within the past month
- History of tick bite, esp. within past 2 weeks (<25%)†
- Late spring or summer (esp. June, July, August)

Rash

- Expanding lesion over days (rather than rapid expansion over hours or stable rash over months)
- Central clearing (37%) or target appearance†
- Minimal pruritus or tenderness
- Central papular erythema, pigmentation or scaling at the site of the tick bite (punctum)
- Lack of scaling (except at the center of the rash, in fading rashes of long duration, or after treatment with antibiotics or topical corticosteroids)
- Location at sites unusual for bacterial cellulitis (e.g., axillae, popliteal fossae, groin, waist)

Associated Symptoms†

- Fatigue (54%)
- Myalgia/Arthralgia (44%)
- Headache (42%)
- Fever and/or chills (39%)
- Stiff neck (35%)
  (Respiratory and gastrointestinal complaints are infrequent)

Physical Examination

- Regional lymphadenopathy (23%)
- Fever (16%)

*Not meant to be restrictive; exceptions occur.
†Percentages refer to our experience in culture-confirmed patients (28).
Reprinted with permission from Nadelman RB, Wormser GP. Erythema migrans and early Lyme disease. Am J Med 1995;98(suppl 4A):15S-24S.

veillance definition for EM. Such rapidly developing EM-like rashes that are not associated with systemic symptoms may often be safely observed for 24 to 48 hours. Spontaneous resolution within this time suggests a local reaction to an arthropod bite rather than EM (see Case 3.2). Persistence or expansion of the rash and/or the development of systemic symptoms should suggest the diagnosis of EM (or of a local pyogenic infection at the site of the tick bite) and the need for antibiotic treatment.

Table 3.3   Differential Diagnosis of Erythema Migrans in the United States*

Disorders (Other Than EM)	Characteristics Distinguishing the Disorder from EM
Disorders occurring year-round	
Bacterial cellulitis (streptococcal or staphylococcal)	Sudden onset; predisposing risk factor (e.g., abnormal vasculature, diabetes mellitus); presence on lower extremities; lymphangitis; high fever and leukocytosis common
Tinea	Thin raised borders with scaling; absence of systemic symptoms; stable size for weeks to months; positive KOH preparation
Granuloma annulare	Dermal papules (or subcutaneous lesions) that spread over weeks to months; may be present for years; usually <5 cm; most common on dorsum of hands or feet; multiple rings occurring symmetrically
Erythema annulare centrifugum	Indistinct border with scaling and pruritus or firm indurated gyrate border; underlying disease process (e.g., neoplasm, infection, drug reaction) may be present
Urticaria	Predisposing factor (e.g., medication history); raised lesions; prominent pruritus; absence of systemic symptoms; sudden appearance and evanescence
Erythema multiforme	Predisposing factor (e.g., medication history, mycoplasma or herpes simplex infection); may appear on palms and soles and mucous membranes; absence of larger primary lesion; absence of central papules in lesions
Fixed drug reaction	Medication history; appears on face or genitals; prominent burning sensation
Disorders occurring during late spring and summer	
Localized tick bite reaction	Occurs hours after bite (tick may still be attached); often <5 cm; expands over hours; resolves within <48 h; not associated with systemic symptoms
Reaction to insect or spider bite	Bite often recalled by patient; reaction may develop minutes to hours after bite; occurs at exposed areas of the body (e.g., forearm, hand, ankle); significant pruritus or tenderness common; absence of systemic symptoms (except for certain spider bites—e.g., brown recluse spider)
Plant dermatitis (poison ivy/poison oak)	Explosive onset of rash within 6–12 h after contact; edema, severe pruritus, vesiculation common; streaking along the area of contact; occurs on exposed areas of the body (e.g., distal extremities, and face)

*Not meant to be restrictive; exceptions occur. European EM may differ in some ways (e.g., duration).
EM = erythema migrans; KOH = potassium hydroxide.

CASE 3.2 *Tick bite reaction*

A 36-year-old woman presents with a small, slightly pruritic "bull's eye" lesion on her left calf. She first noticed the lesion the same morning, one day after removing an adult deer tick from her calf while she was apple picking (in October) in an area endemic for Lyme disease. The lesion, which appears at the site of the bite, measures 3 cm and is slightly raised with central clearing. She has no other skin lesions, and the remainder of her physical examination is normal. Antibiotics are not prescribed, and the rash fades over the next 2 days. She remains well.

Insect Bite Reactions

Significant pruritus or tenderness are more typical of arthropod bite reactions than EM. Unlike EM, insect bites tend to occur on exposed body parts, such as the face, forearm, ankle, or hand. In contrast to a tick bite, which is usually asymptomatic, patients may recall the exact moment when a spider or insect bite occurred. Unlike the macular or minimally raised lesions of EM, *urticarial* reactions to bites are elevated above normal skin, are pruritic, and resolve in within 24 to 48 hours (72).

Bacterial Cellulitis

In contrast to EM, streptococcal or staphylococcal cellulitis is painful, develops suddenly, and evolves over hours. Lymphangitis may be associated with cellulitis, but does not occur with EM. A predisposing risk factor (diabetes mellitus, peripheral vascular disease, tinea pedis, or previous surgery or trauma) is often present. Rigors, leukocytosis, and a toxic-appearing state suggest cellulitis rather than Lyme disease. Bacterial cellulitis occurs most commonly on the distal lower extremities, unlike EM lesions, which are more likely to occur proximally (e.g., on the popliteal fossae, thighs, shoulders, axillae, or groin) or on the trunk.

Tinea

Like EM, tinea appears as annular lesions with erythematous borders, often with central clearing (73). However, the presence of scale, a thin raised border, or psoriasiform lesion, should suggest tinea (73). Erythema migrans is less likely than tinea to be bilateral and symmetric. Brightly erythematous plaques in the groin with peripheral satellite pustules should suggest candidiasis (73). A potassium hydroxide (KOH) preparation of a skin scraping may reveal fungal forms, supporting the diagnosis of candida or tinea.

Plant Dermatitis

Plant dermatitis (e.g., poison ivy and poison oak) is one of the most common causes of allergic contact dermatitis in North America (74), and may resemble EM, particularly after application of topical corticosteroids. A history of exposure may be helpful in making the diagnosis. An explosive onset of rash (within 6 to 12 hours after contact in those who are exquisitely sensitive), associated with edema, vesiculation, and marked pruritus, is most suggestive of plant dermatitis (74). Rashes on exposed body areas, such as the distal extremities and face, are more typical of plant dermatitis than EM (75).

Miscellaneous Causes

Erythema multiforme and urticaria may appear similar to multiple EM lesions. However, the former lack the central papular erythema or postinflammatory skin change seen with the larger primary lesion of EM. In contrast to EM, the presence of pruritus is typical of urticaria and erythema multiforme may involve the palms and soles. Skin biopsy may help clarify the diagnosis in difficult cases. Granuloma annulare (76), erythema annulare centrifugum (77), and fixed drug reactions (78) may occasionally be confused with EM (see Table 3.3).

Viral-like Illnesses Without Rash

Evaluation for a "viral" illness during the late spring and summer should include a complete skin examination, with all clothes removed, in order to detect an EM lesion that may be unrecognized by the patient. Other tick-borne illnesses in endemic areas, such as Rocky Mountain spotted fever, babesiosis, ehrlichiosis, and tick-borne encephalitis (in Europe), as well as enteroviral infections, may need to be considered.

Human granulocytic ehrlichiosis may be particularly difficult to distinguish from early Lyme disease, because fever with headache, myalgia, and malaise may occur with both infections and because human granulocytic ehrlichiosis appears to be associated with false-positive ELISA and Western immunoblot assays for *B. burgdorferi* (79). Reports of concurrent Lyme disease and babesiosis (80) or ehrlichiosis (44) confound matters further because all three infections are transmitted by *I. scapularis*. Helpful laboratory tests include 1) examination of the peripheral blood smear for intraerythrocytic parasite forms in babesiosis or for leukocytic inclusions (morulae) in ehrlichiosis; and 2) a complete blood count (thrombocytopenia, anemia, or leukopenia commonly occur with babesiosis and ehrlichiosis, whereas the complete blood count in patients with Lyme disease is typically normal [63]).

Treatment of Early Lyme Disease

General Considerations

A 10- to 21-day course of any of a number of β-lactam or tetracycline antimicrobials is effective in the treatment of EM and its associated symptoms

(Box 3.2) (81). Because EM resolves spontaneously, drug efficacy cannot be measured solely by disappearance of the rash. Patients with objective evidence of arthritis, meningitis, and carditis after receiving treatment for EM can be considered treatment failures. However, such cases occur infrequently. Thus, large multi-center studies are required to detect small differences in clinical activity (81,82).

The efficacy of oral antibiotics in the treatment of EM and associated signs and symptoms is noteworthy (32,53,54,82), despite the low levels many of these drugs attain in the central nervous system, where spirochetes may spread soon after infection (83). In one study, treatment failures were more likely to occur in patients presenting with dysesthesia (54). However, evidence from a recent large multicenter trial indicated that even patients with proven disseminated early disease do equally well with treatment with oral doxycycline or intravenous ceftriaxone (84).

Recommended Antibiotics

A variety of oral drugs—including amoxicillin, penicillin, tetracycline, doxycycline, and cefuroxime axetil—are effective in hastening the resolution of EM and its associated symptoms and in preventing extracutaneous complications (Table 3.4) (81,85,86).

Although amoxicillin and doxycycline may have pharmacokinetic advantages over penicillin and tetracycline, respectively (88), there is no evidence that they are superior clinically. One retrospective study found tetracycline and doxycycline to have similar efficacy (89).

Box 3.2   Recommendations for Treatment of Early Lyme Disease

1. Treatment is indicated for all patients with erythema migrans (EM) rash with or without associated symptoms.
2. Testing blood for antibodies to *Borrelia burgdorferi* is not necessary to confirm the diagnosis of EM, and has no role in monitoring response to treatment.
3. Empiric treatment may be considered for *selected* patients who have a small (<5 cm) rash, especially if it is associated with systemic symptoms suggestive of Lyme disease.
4. Patients who develop a febrile illness without rash during the summer or late spring may be considered for empiric treatment using a tetracycline to provide broader coverage against other potential pathogens (e.g., agents of ehrlichiosis and Rocky Mountain spotted fever).
5. Oral doxycycline, 100 mg twice daily, or amoxicillin, 500 mg three times daily, should be considered the first-line drugs for treating early Lyme disease.
6. Women who develop EM during pregnancy may be considered for treatment with intravenous penicillin or ceftriaxone, although it has not been established that these agents are more effective than oral amoxicillin.

Table 3.4   Oral Treatment of Early Lyme Disease Associated with Erythema Migrans*†

Treatment	Antimicrobial Agent‡	Adult Dosage	Pediatric Dosages§
First Line	Doxycycline‖	100 mg bid	(see footnote)‖
	Amoxicillin	500 mg tid	40–50 mg/kg/d ÷ tid
Alternatives	Phenoxymethyl penicillin	500 mg qid	50 mg/kg/d ÷ tid–qid
	Tetracycline‖	500 mg qid	(see footnote)‖
	Cefuroxime axetil¶	500 mg bid	30 mg/kg/d ÷ bid
Second Line	Azithromycin#	500 mg once daily	5–12 mg/kg (once daily)
	Erythromycin	500 mg qid	30–40 mg/kg/d ÷ qid
	Clarithromycin**	500 mg bid	15 mg/kg/d ÷ bid

*Published clinical experience is mostly limited to adult patients.
†EM patients with extracutaneous disease (e.g., advanced heart block or meningitis) should be treated with IV ceftriaxone (2 g/d) or penicillin G (20 million U daily).
‡The optimum duration of treatment has not been established, but 10 to 30 days of treatment has been recommended (85). Our standard regimen is 14 days.
§Not to exceed adult dosage; dosage is based upon *Red Book* [84] or package insert; consult package insert for safety limitations.
‖Not recommended for children <9 years old or during pregnancy or lactation; for children ≥9 years old, doxycycline dose is 2–4 mg/kg/d ÷ bid and tetracycline dose is 25–50 mg/kg/d ÷ qid.
¶Cefuroxime axetil is the only drug to be granted FDA approval for the treatment of Lyme disease.
#Azithromycin has been given for 5 to 10 days as treatment for EM in adults (55,82).
**The only published clinical study (patients ≥16 years old) was a small, open-label, noncomparison trial (87).
Adapted with permission from Nadelman RB, Wormser GP. Erythema migrans and early Lyme disease. Am J Med. 1995;98(suppl 4A):15S-24S.

Formal approval by the Food and Drug Administration has been granted only to cefuroxime axetil for treatment of Lyme disease. However, first-generation cephalosporins, such as cephalexin, should *not* be used to treat Lyme disease in view of their poor *in vitro* activity and because there have been a number of documented treatment failures (90). Other oral cephalosporins have not been studied sufficiently for their use in the treatment of Lyme disease to be recommended.

Erythromycin has been recommended as an alternative agent for patients who cannot tolerate penicillins or tetracyclines. However, erythromycin was no more effective than no treatment in shortening EM duration and tended to be less effective than tetracycline ($P < 0.07$) in preventing certain extracutaneous complications after EM (91). Azithromycin was significantly less effective than amoxicillin in a large multicenter treatment trial, despite its excellent *in vitro* activity (82). Clarithromycin is also highly effective *in vitro* and in an animal model against *B. burgdorferi* (92), but it has been studied clinically in only one preliminary uncontrolled treatment trial (87).

In view of the described experience (and that for roxithromycin, which had disappointing results in a European study [93]), the use of any of the macrolide drugs in early Lyme disease as first-line therapy cannot be recommended.

Quinolones have no appreciable activity against *B. burgdorferi* (they are sometimes used in *Borrelia* culture media [49,58]).

Treatment During Pregnancy

Early Lyme disease during pregnancy has been associated with fetal morbidity and mortality (40–42). At least one neonatal death has been linked to transplacental spirochete transmission in a pregnant European woman even though she received oral penicillin treatment for EM during the first trimester (41). Intravenous penicillin or ceftriaxone has sometimes been recommended for EM occurring during gestation. Clinical superiority of parenteral treatment compared with oral therapy has not been demonstrated in this setting.

Treatment Duration

Many physicians prescribe several weeks of an oral antibiotic for patients with EM. However, the only published prospective trial addressing the effect of varying durations of oral antimicrobials failed to detect a difference between patients who received tetracycline for 10 days and those who received tetracycline for 20 days (94). Outcome at 1 year was similar in a separate retrospective study comparing patients who received doxycycline for 14 days and those who received the same antibiotic for 20 days (89). It is our practice to treat most patients with EM for 2 weeks.

Empiric Therapy in the Absence of a Definite EM Lesion

Patients in endemic areas with febrile, viral-like syndromes occurring in the late spring and summer may sometimes warrant empiric treatment for Lyme disease. Small (<5 cm) rashes that resemble EM but do not fulfill CDC criteria may also merit empiric treatment if associated with systemic symptoms suggestive of Lyme disease. Serial assays for antibody to *B. burgdorferi* may help confirm the clinical diagnosis of Lyme disease.

Use of a tetracycline for illnesses suggestive of early Lyme disease but without rash has the important advantage of providing antimicrobial coverage for the rickettsial agents of Rocky Mountain spotted fever and ehrlichiosis. It is our practice to give amoxicillin-clavulanate (500 mg three times daily) or cefuroxime axetil to patients in whom EM cannot be distinguished from bacterial cellulitis, in order to include antimicrobial coverage against streptococci and staphylococci as well as against *B. burgdorferi*.

Prognosis

In patients with EM who receive appropriate courses of antimicrobial therapy (see Table 3.4), the rash and fever (if present) improve rapidly. EM rashes resolve spontaneously (without treatment) within a median of 28 days.

Persistence of *B. burgdorferi* at the site of EM after the completion of antibiotic treatment has been reported anecdotally in a small group of European patients (94). However, two separate prospective studies in the United States failed to confirm this observation (51,95). The disparate results in the European and North American studies may be attributed to the different virulence characteristics of the different *Borrelia* spp. seen on the two continents (Strle and colleagues, unpublished data, 1997).

Serologic assays may remain positive for years after successful resolution of early Lyme disease (96) and are not recommended for follow-up after treatment. EM does not appear to confer lasting immunity to Lyme disease. Reinfection with *B. burgdorferi*, as manifested by a second EM at a different site, has been documented by culture (97).

Objective evidence of treatment failure is uncommon after antimicrobial therapy for EM (32,54,55). However, some patients develop fibromyalgia (98) or "post-Lyme" syndrome manifested principally by arthralgia and fatigue of uncertain origin (*see* Chapter 8, "Long-Term Consequences of Lyme Disease") (99). Retreatment in these patients has not been beneficial in anecdotal reports (98,100). Cognitive defects have been identified (in a retrospective study) in some patients after treatment for early Lyme disease (101). However, many of these patients had substantial treatment delays (several years) or did not receive currently recommended antibiotic regimens. In addition, patients with preexisting cognitive problems (unrelated to Lyme disease) were not excluded.

Diagnosis should be re-evaluated in patients who fail to respond to treatment for EM and associated symptoms. The most important reason for treatment failure is erroneous diagnosis (e.g., tinea). Other possible explanations may include poor compliance with treatment and coinciding tickborne disorders (including babesiosis and ehrlichiosis). Some patients with EM who have early unrecognized central nervous system disease may also have incomplete improvement. The role of post-infectious phenomena causing symptoms after spirochete eradication is discussed elsewhere (*see* Chapter 5, "Neurologic Manifestations of Lyme Disease," and Chapter 8, "Long-Term Consequences of Lyme Disease").

■ ■ ■

Key Points

• Incidence of Lyme disease is less than 5% after an *Ixodes scapularis* bite.

• Prophylactic antibiotics are not presently recommended after a tick bite because efficacy has not been demonstrated and because of the risk of adverse effects.

• Clinicians may choose to treat asymptomatic pregnant women who have been bitten by an *I. scapularis* nymph or adult tick prophylactically with oral amoxicillin (for approximately 10 days).

• The erythema migrans rash, which occurs within a mean of 7 to 10 days after a tick bite, is present in 90% or more of patients with objective evidence of Lyme disease.

• Drugs of choice for treating erythema migrans in adults are oral doxycycline or amoxicillin. Cefuroxime axetil can be used as an alternative.

Acknowledgments.   We thank the staff of the Lyme Disease Diagnostic Center at the Westchester County Medical Center for their tireless efforts, and our patients for their participation in the research protocols.

Drs. Nadelman and Wormser are supported in part by grants from the National Institute of Arthritis and Musculoskeletal and Skin Diseases (RO1-AR41508 [RBN, GPW] and RO1-AR43135 [GPW]), and from the Centers for Disease Control and Prevention (CDC) (Cooperative Agreements U50/CCU 210286 [RBN] and U50/CCU 210280 [GPW]). Dr. Nadelman is also supported in part by a grant from the New York State Department of Health, Tick-Borne Disease Institute (C-011001). The contents of this report are solely the responsibility of the authors and do not necessarily represent the official views of any of the above agencies.

Parts of this chapter were adapted from an article that appeared in the *American Journal of Medicine* (1995;89[Suppl 4A]:15S-24S) and appear with permission of Excerpta Medica, Inc.

■ ■ ■

REFERENCES

1. **Needham GR.** Evaluation of five popular methods for tick removal. Pediatrics. 1985;75:997-1002.

2. **Fish D.** Environmental risk and prevention of Lyme disease. Am J Med. 1995;98(Suppl 4A):2S-9S.

3. **Matuschka F-R, Spielman A.** The vector of the Lyme disease spirochete. N Engl J Med. 1992;327:542.

4. **Saltzman MB, Rubin LG, Sood SK.** Prevention of Lyme disease after tick bites [letter]. N Engl J Med. 1993;328:137.

5. **Sood SK, Salzman MB, Johnson BJB, et al.** Duration of tick attachment as a predictor of the risk of Lyme disease in an area in which Lyme disease is endemic. J Infect Dis. 1997;175:996-9.

6. **Barbour AG, Maupin GO, Teltow GJ, et al.** Identification of an uncultivable *Borrelia* species in the hard tick *Amblyomma americanum*: possible agent of a Lyme disease-like illness. J Infect Dis. 1996;173:403-9.

7. **McDade JE, Newhouse VF.** Natural history of *Rickettsia rickettsii*. Annu Rev Microbiol. 1986;40:287-309.

8. **Campbell GL, Paul WS, Schriefer ME, et al.** Epidemiologic and diagnostic studies of patients with suspected early Lyme disease, Missouri, 1990–1993. J Infect Dis. 1995;172:470-80.

9. **Falco RC, Fish D.** Ticks parasitizing humans in a Lyme disease endemic area of southern New York State. Am J Epidemiol. 1988;128:1146-52.

10. **Costello CM, Steere AC, Pinkerton RE, Feder HM Jr.** A prospective study of tick bites in an endemic area for Lyme disease. J Infect Dis. 1989;159:136-9.

11. **Shapiro ED, Gerber MA, Holabird NB, et al.** A controlled trial of antimicrobial prophylaxis for Lyme disease after deer-tick bites. N Engl J Med. 1992;327:1769-73.

12. **Agre F, Schwartz R.** The value of early treatment of deer tick bite for the prevention of Lyme disease. Am J Dis Child. 1993;147:945-7.

13. **Nadelman RB, Forseter G, Horowitz H, et al.** Natural history of patients bitten by *Ixodes dammini (Id)* in Westchester County, New York, USA [abstract]. In: Proceedings and abstracts of the Fifth International Conference on Lyme Borreliosis, Washington, D.C. May 30–June 2, 1992. Bethesda, MD: Federation of American Societies for Experimental Biology, 1992:A80.

14. **Magid D, Schwartz B, Craft J, Schwartz JS.** Prevention of Lyme disease after tick bites: a cost-effectiveness analysis. N Engl J Med. 1992;327:534-41.

15. **Maupin GO, Fish D, Zultowsky J, et al.** Landscape ecology of Lyme disease in a residential area of Westchester County, New York. Am J Epidemiol. 1991;133:1105-13.

16. **Olson PE, Richards AL, Dasch GA, Kennedy CA.** Failure to identify *Borrelia burgdorferi* in southern California by DNA amplification [letter]. J Infect Dis. 1993;168:257-8.

17. **Magnarelli LA, Anderson JF, Fish D.** Transovarial transmission of *Borrelia burgdorferi* in *Ixodes dammini* (Acari:Ixodidae). J Infect Dis. 1987;156:234-6.

18. **Schwartz BS, Ribeiro JMC, Goldstein MD.** Anti-tick antibodies: an epidemiologic tool in Lyme disease research. Am J Epidemiol. 1990;132:58-66.

19. **Hofmeister EK, Childs JE.** Analysis of *Borrelia burgdorferi* sequentially isolated from *Peromyscus leucopus* captured at a Lyme disease enzootic site. J Infect Dis. 1995;172:462-9.

20. **Johnson WD Jr.** *Borrelia* species (relapsing fever). In: Mandell GL, Bennett JE, Dolin R, eds. Principles and Practice of Infectious Diseases. 4th ed. New York: Churchill Livingstone; 1995:2141-3.

21. **Piesman J.** Dynamics of *Borrelia burgdorferi* transmission by nymphal *Ixodes dammini* ticks. J Infect Dis. 1993;167:1082-5.

22. **Klempner MS, Noring R, Epstein B, et al.** Binding of human plasminogen and urokinase-type plasminogen activator to the Lyme disease spirochete, *Borrelia burgdorferi.* J Infect Dis. 1995;171:1258-65.

23. **Shih C-M, Spielman A.** Accelerated transmission of Lyme disease spirochetes by partially fed vector ticks. J Clin Microbiol. 1993;2878-81.

24. **Schwartz B, Nadelman RB, Fish D, et al.** Entomologic and demographic correlates of anti-tick saliva antibody in a prospective study of tick bite subjects in Westchester County, New York. Am J Trop Med Hyg. 1993;48:50-7.

25. **Falco RC, Fish D, Piesman J.** Duration of tick bites in a Lyme-endemic area. Am J Epidemiol. 1996;143:187-92.

26. **Schwartz I, Varde S, Nadelman RB, et al.** Inhibition of efficient polymerase chain reaction amplification of *Borrelia burgdorferi* DNA in blood-fed ticks. Am J Trop Med Hyg. 1997;56:339-42.

27. **Berger BW.** Dermatologic manifestations of Lyme disease. Rev Infect Dis. 1989;11:S1475-81.

28. **Nadelman RB, Nowakowski J, Forseter G, et al.** The clinical spectrum of early Lyme borreliosis in patients with culture confirmed erythema migrans. Am J Med. 1996;100:502-8.

29. **Melski JW, Reed KD, Mitchell PD, Barth GD.** Primary and secondary erythema migrans in central Wisconsin. Arch Dermatol. 1993;129:709-16.

30. **Steere AC, Bartenhagen NH, Craft JE, et al.** The early clinical manifestations of Lyme disease. Ann Intern Med. 1983;99:76-82.

31. **Warshafsky S, Nowakowski J, Nadelman RB, et al.** Efficacy of antibiotic prophylaxis for prevention of Lyme disease: a meta-analysis. J Gen Intern Med. 1996;11:329 33.

32. **Nadelman RB, Luger SW, Frank E, et al.** Comparison of cefuroxime axetil and doxycycline in the treatment of early Lyme disease. Ann Intern Med. 1992;117:273-80.

33. **Campbell GL, Fritz CL, Fish D, et al.** An algebraic model for estimating the annual frequency of *Ixodes scapularis* bites in human populations [Abstract]. Proceedings of the Seventh International Conference on Lyme borreliosis; June 16-21, 1996; San Francisco.

34. **Shih CM, Spielman A.** Topical prophylaxis for Lyme disease after tick bite in a rodent model. J Infect Dis. 1993;168:1042-5.

35. **Steere AC, Taylor E, Wilson ML, et al.** Longitudinal assessment of the clinical and epidemiologic features of Lyme disease in a defined population. J Infect Dis. 1986;154:295-300.

36. **Steere AC.** Lyme disease. N Engl J Med. 1989;321:586-96.

37. **Gerber MA, Shapiro ED, Burke GS, et al.** Lyme disease in children in southeastern Connecticut. N Engl J Med. 1996;335:1270-4.

38. **Wormser GP, McKenna D, Nadelman RB, et al.** Lyme disease in children [letter]. N Engl J Med. 1997;336:1107.

39. **Kassirer JP.** Is a tick's bark worse than its bite? Formulating an answer with decision analysis. N Engl J Med. 1992;327:562-3.

40. **Markowitz LE, Steere AC, Benach JL, et al.** Lyme disease during pregnancy. JAMA. 1986;255:3394-6.

41. **Weber K, Bratzke H, Neubert U, et al.** *Borrelia burgdorferi* in a newborn despite oral penicillin for Lyme borreliosis during pregnancy. Pediatr Infect Dis J. 1988;7:286-9.

42. **Maraspin V, Cimperman J, Lotrič-Furlan S, et al.** Treatment of erythema migrans in pregnancy. Clin Infect Dis. 1996;22:788-93.

43. **Pancholi P, Kolbert C, Mitchell PD, et al.** *Ixodes dammini* as a potential vector of human granulocytic ehrlichiosis. J Infect Dis. 1995;172:1007-12.

44. **Nadelman RB, Horowitz HW, Hsieh TC, et al.** Simultaneous human granulocytic ehrlichiosis and Lyme borreliosis. N Engl J Med. 1997;337:27-30.

45. **Malane MS, Grant-Kels JM, Feder HM Jr, Luger SW.** Diagnosis of Lyme disease based on dermatologic manifestations. Ann Intern Med. 1991;114:490-8.

46. **Nadelman RB, Wormser GP.** Erythema migrans and early Lyme disease. Am J Med. 1995;98(suppl 4A):15S-24S.

47. **Centers for Disease Control.** Case definitions for public health surveillance. MMWR Morb Mortal Wkly Rep. 1990;39(no. RR-13):19-21.

48. **Åsbrink E, Olsson I.** Clinical manifestations of erythema chronicum migrans Afzelius in 161 patients. Acta Derm Venereol (Stockh) 1985;65:43-52.

49. **Berger BW, Johnson RC, Kodner C, Coleman L.** Cultivation of *Borrelia burgdorferi* from erythema migrans lesions and perilesional skin. J Clin Microbiol. 1992;30:359-61.

50. **Wormser GP, Forseter G, Cooper D, et al.** Use of a novel technique of cutaneous lavage for diagnosis of Lyme disease associated with erythema migrans. JAMA. 1992;268:1311-3.

51. **Nadelman RB, Nowakowski J, Forseter G, et al.** Failure to isolate *Borrelia burgdorferi* after antimicrobial therapy in culture-documented Lyme borreliosis associated with erythema migrans: report of a prospective study. Am J Med. 1993;94:583-8.

52. **Goldberg NS, Forseter G, Nadelman RB, et al.** Vesicular erythema migrans. Arch Dermatol. 1992;128:1495-8.

53. **Dattwyler RJ, Volkman DJ, Conaty SM, et al.** Amoxycillin plus probenecid versus doxycycline for treatment of erythema migrans borreliosis. Lancet. 1990; 336:1404-6.

54. **Massarotti EM, Luger SW, Rahn DW, et al.** Treatment of early Lyme disease. Am J Med. 1992;92:396-403.

55. **Weber K, Wilske B, Preac-Mursic V, Thurmayr R.** Azithromycin versus penicillin V for the treatment of early Lyme borreliosis. Infection. 1993;21:367-72.

56. **Williams CL, Strobino B, Lee A, et al.** Lyme disease in childhood: clinical and epidemiologic features of ninety cases. Pediatr Infect Dis. 1990;9:10-4.

57. **Steere AC, Schoen RT, Taylor E.** The clinical evolution of Lyme arthritis. Ann Intern Med. 1987;107:725-31.

58. **Nadelman RB, Pavia CS, Magnarelli LA, Wormser GP.** Isolation of *Borrelia burgdorferi* from the blood of seven patients with Lyme disease. Am J Med. 1990;88:21-6.

59. **Feder HM Jr, Gerber MA, Krause PJ, et al.** Early Lyme disease: a flu-like illness without erythema migrans. Pediatrics. 1993;91:456-9.

60. **Shrestha M, Grodzicki RL, Steere AC.** Diagnosing early Lyme disease. Am J Med. 1985;78:235-240.

61. **Berardi VP, Weeks KE, Steere AC.** Serodiagnosis of early Lyme disease: analysis of IgM and IgG antibody responses by using an antibody-capture enzyme immunoassay. J Infect Dis. 1988;158:754-60.

62. **Aguero-Rosenfeld M, Nowakowski J, McKenna DF, et al.** Serodiagnosis in early Lyme disease. J Clin Microbiol. 1993;31:3090-5.

63. **Nadelman RB, Strle F, Horowitz HW, et al.** Leukopenia, thrombocytopenia, and Lyme borreliosis: is there an association? [Letter]. Clin Infect Dis. 1997;24:1027-8.

64. **Rubin DA, Sorbera C, Nikitin P, et al.** Prospective evaluation of heart block complicating early Lyme disease. Pacing Clin Electrophysiol 1992;15:252-5.

65. **van Dam AP, Kuiper H, Vos K, et al.** Different genospecies of *Borrelia burgdorferi* are associated with distinct clinical manifestations of Lyme borreliosis. Clin Infect Dis. 1993;17:708-17.

66. **Pollack RJ, Telford SR III, Spielman A.** Standardization for culturing Lyme disease spirochetes. J Clin Microbiol. 1993;31:1251-5.

67. **Nadelman RB, Schwartz I, Wormser GP.** Detecting *Borrelia burgdorferi* in blood from patients with Lyme disease. [Letter]. J Infect Dis. 1994;169:1410-1.

68. **Goodman JL, Bradley JF, Ross AE, et al.** Bloodstream invasion in early Lyme disease: results from a prospective, controlled, blinded study using the polymerase chain reaction. Am J Med. 1995;99:6-12.

69. **Wormser GP, Nowakowski J, Nadelman RB, et al.** Improving the yield of blood cultures in early Lyme disease. J Clin Microbiol. (In Press).

70. **Schwartz I, Wormser GP, Schwartz JJ, et al.** Diagnosis of early Lyme disease by polymerase chain reaction amplification and culture of skin biopsies from erythema migrans lesions. J Clin Microbiol. 1992;30:3082-8.

71. **Feder HM Jr, Whitaker DL.** Misdiagnosis of erythema migrans. Am J Med. 1995;99:412-9.

72. **Soter NA.** Urticaria and angioedema. In: Fitzpatrick TB, Eisen AZ, Wolff K, et al, eds. Dermatology in General Medicine. 4th ed. New York: McGraw-Hill; 1993:1483-94.

73. **Martin AG, Kobayashi GS.** Superficial fungal infection: dermatophytosis, tinca, nigra, piedra. In: Fitzpatrick TB, Eisen AZ, Wolff K, et al, eds. Dermatology in General Medicine. 4th ed. New York: McGraw-Hill; 1993:2421-51.

74. **Epstein WL.** Allergic contact dermatitis. In: Fitzpatrick TB, Eisen AZ, Wolff K, et al, eds. Dermatology in General Medicine. 3rd ed. New York: McGraw-Hill; 1987: 1373-83.

75. **Goldschmidt H, Grekin RC, eds.** Contact dermatitis: drug eruptions. In: Andrews' Diseases of the Skin Clinical Dermatology. 8th ed. Philadelphia: WB Saunders; 1990:89-130.

76. **Dahl MV.** Granuloma annulare. In: Fitzpatrick TB, Eisen AZ, Wolff K, et al, eds. Dermatology in General Medicine. 4th ed. New York: McGraw-Hill; 1993:1187-91.

77. **Burgdorf WHC.** In: Fitzpatrick TB, Eisen AZ, Wolff K, et al, eds. Dermatology in General Medicine. 4th ed. New York: McGraw-Hill; 1993:1183-6.

78. **Blacker KL, Stern RS, Wintroub BU.** Cutaneous reactions to drugs. In: Fitzpatrick TB, Eisen AZ, Wolff K, et al, eds. Dermatology in General Medicine. 4th ed. New York: McGraw-Hill; 1993:1783-95.

79. **Wormser GP, Horowitz HW, Dumler JS, et al.** False-positive Lyme serology in human granulocyte ehrlichiosis [letter]. Lancet. 1996;347:981-2.

80. **Marcus LC, Steere AC, Duray PH, et al.** Fatal pancarditis in a patient with coexistent Lyme disease and babesiosis: demonstration of spirochetes in the myocardium. Ann Intern Med. 1985;103:374-6.

81. **Wormser GP.** Lyme disease: insights into the use of antimicrobials for prevention and treatment in the context of experience with other spirochetal infections. Mt Sinai J Med. 1995;62:188-95.

82. **Luft BJ, Dattwyler RJ, Johnson RC, et al.** Azithromycin compared with amoxicillin in the treatment of erythema migrans: a double-blind randomized, controlled trial. Ann Intern Med. 1996;124:785-91.

83. **Luft BJ, Steinman CR, Neimark HC, et al.** Invasion of the central nervous system by *Borrelia burgdorferi* in acute disseminated infection. JAMA. 1992;267: 1364-7.

84. **Dattwyler RJ, Luft BJ, Kunkel MJ, et al.** Ceftriaxone compared with doxycycline for the treatment of acute disseminate Lyme disease. N Engl J Med. 1997;337:289-94.

85. Treatment of Lyme disease. Med Lett Drugs Ther. 1992;34:95-7.

86. **American Academy of Pediatrics.** Committee on Infectious Diseases. Section 5: Antimicrobials and related therapy. In: Peter G, ed. 1994 Red Book: Report of the Committee on Infectious Diseases. 23rd ed. Elk Grove Village, IL: American Academy of Pediatrics; 1994:541-57.

87. **Dattwyler RJ, Grunwaldt E, Luft BJ.** Clarithromycin in treatment of early Lyme disease: a pilot study. Antimicrob Agents Chemother. 1996;40:468-9.

88. **Neu HC.** A perspective on therapy of Lyme infection. Am N Y Acad Sci. 1988;539:314-6.

89. **Nowakowski J, Nadelman RB, Forseter G, et al.** Doxycycline versus tetracycline therapy for Lyme disease associated with erythema migrans. J Am Acad Dermatol. 1995;32:223-7.

90. **Nowakowski J, McKenna DF, Nadelman RB, et al.** Culture-confirmed treatment failures of cephalexin therapy for erythema migrans [Abstract]. Seventh International Conference on Lyme Borreliosis, San Francisco, CA, June 16-21, 1996.

91. **Steere AC, Hutchinson GJ, Rahn DW, et al.** Treatment of the early manifestations of Lyme disease. Ann Intern Med. 1983;99:22-6.

92. **Alder J, Mitten M, Jarvis K, et al.** Efficacy of clarithromycin for treatment of experimental Lyme disease *in vivo*. Antimicrob Agents Chemother. 1993;37:1329-33.

93. **Hansen K, Hovmark A, Lebech A-M, et al.** Roxithromycin in Lyme borreliosis: discrepant results of an *in vitro* and *in vivo* aimal susceptibility study and a clinical trial in patients with erythema migrans. Acta Derma Venereol. 1991;72:297-300.

94. **Preac-Mursic V, Weber K, Pfister HW, et al.** Survival of *Borrelia burgdorferi* in antibiotically treated patients with Lyme borreliosis. Infection. 1989;17:355-9.

95. **Berger BW, Johnson RC, Kodner C, Coleman L.** Failure of *Borrelia burgdorferi* to survive in the skin of patients with antibiotic-treated Lyme disease. J Am Acad Dermatol. 1992;27:34-7.

96. **Feder HM, Gerber MA, Luger SW, Ryan RW.** Persistence of antibodies to *Borrelia burgdorferi* in patients treated for Lyme disease. Clin Infect Dis. 1992;15:788-93.

97. **Nowakowski J, Schwartz I, Nadelman RB, et al.** Culture-confirmed infection and reinfection with *Borrelia burgdorferi*. Ann Intern Med. 1997. (In press).

98. **Dinerman H, Steere AC.** Lyme disease associated with fibromyalgia. Ann Intern Med. 1992;117:281-5.

99. **Sigal LH.** Persisting complaints attributed to chronic Lyme disease: possible mechanisms and implications for management. Am J Med. 1994;96:365-74.

100. **Steere AC, Taylor E, McHugh GL, Logigian EL.** The overdiagnosis of Lyme disease. JAMA. 1993;269:1812-16.

101. **Shadick NA, Phillips CB, Logigian EL, et al.** The long-term clinical outcome of Lyme disease. A population-based retrospective cohort study. Ann Intern Med. 1994;121:560-7.

KEY REFERENCES

Fish D. Environmental risk and prevention of Lyme disease. Am J Med. 1995;98(suppl 4A):2S-9S.

Excellent description of Ixodes scapularis *and its role in transmitting Lyme disease.*

Nadelman RB, Nowakowski RB, Forseter G, et al. The clinical spectrum of early Lyme borreliosis in patients with culture-confirmed erythema migrans. Am J Med. 1996;100:502-8.

The largest series of patients with EM in the United States in whom the diagnosis was established by isolating Borrelia burgdorferi *from clinical specimens.*

Shapiro ED, Gerber MA, Holabird NB, et al. A controlled trial of antimicrobial prophylaxis for Lyme disease after deer-tick bites. N Engl J Med. 1992;327:1769-73.

Reports that amoxicillin prophylaxis after a tick bite was no more effective than placebo in preventing Lyme disease. The largest published clinical trial in the United States to date.

Steere AC, Bartenhagen NH, Craft JE, et al. The early clinical manifestations of Lyme disease. Ann Intern Med. 1983;99:76-82.

The landmark paper summarizing the findings of more than 300 patients with erythema migrans.

Wormser GP. Lyme disease: insights into the use of antimicrobials for prevention and treatment in the context of experience with other spirochetal infections. Mt Sinai J Med. 1995;62:188-95.

Overview of many of the issues related to the choice and duration of antibiotic treatment of tick bites and early Lyme disease.

4

■ ■ ■

Lyme Carditis

Janine Evans, MD

Lyme carditis complicates infection with *Borrelia burgdorferi* in 4% to 10% of untreated persons with erythema migrans. In patients who have received treatment for early Lyme disease, carditis occurs much less frequently.

Epidemiologic data indicate a male preponderance and an average age of 32 years in the United States and 44 years in Europe for acquiring Lyme carditits, although any gender and age group may be affected (2,4). Carditis typically develops within 3 to 5 weeks [range, <1 wk to 7 mo) after the appearance of erythema migrans, during the acute disseminated phase of infection. Although Lyme disease is often accompanied by other clinical features of early infection, heart block can be the sole presenting symptom (2,3). Atrioventricular (AV) conduction disturbances, myocarditis, and pericarditis are the most common manifestations of Lyme carditis (Box 4.1). Chronic dilated cardiomyopathy and other conduction disturbances have also been described. Lyme carditis typically resolves spontaneously without sequelae; however, some patients require temporary pacemakers.

Conduction Abnormalities

Varying degrees of AV block are the most common cardiac abnormality reported to occur in Lyme disease, although myopericarditis, tachyarrhythmias, and cardiac muscle dysfunction may also be present (5). The degree of AV block may fluctuate rapidly, progressing from first-degree to complete heart block and back again in minutes. Patients with complete heart block typically also display first-degree and Wenckebach-type second-degree block.

Box 4.1   Cardiac Manifestations of Lyme Disease

Cardiac conduction defects involving any level of the conducting system
Myocarditis
Pericarditis
Tachyarrhythmias (uncommon)
Chronic cardiomyopathy (?)

In a review of 105 reported cases of Lyme carditis, the distribution of AV block was as follows: 12% first-degree; 16% second-degree; and 49% third-degree heart block (6).

It is likely that many cases of first-degree heart block are undetected because most patients with uncomplicated first-degree heart block do not have symptoms suggestive of cardiac disease. Patients with high-degree heart block are almost always symptomatic. Symptoms include lightheadedness, syncope, dyspnea on exertion, chest pain, and palpitations (see Case 4.1). In Steere and colleagues' (2) original report of 20 patients with Lyme carditis, only 2 of 8 patients with no more than first-degree block had symptoms, and all patients with high-degree heart block had at least one symptom. The most useful clue to cardiac involvement was alternating tachycardia or bradycardia (2). PR intervals greater than 0.3 seconds were identified as the highest risk factor for progression to complete heart block.

Electrocardiographic Patterns

Electrophysiologic studies have demonstrated that the AV node is the most commonly involved site, although all parts of the conduction may be affected (4). Sinoatrial node dysfunction, manifested as sinoatrial node block or abnormalities of nodal recovery time and intra-atrial block, blockage in the His bundles, and combined proximal and distal conduction disturbances have been reported (5,7–9). Supraventricular and ventricular dysrhythmias are uncommon (10).

Escape rhythms are variable. Narrow QRS escape rhythms with reasonable rates typically accompany blocks at or above the level of the AV node and predict a benign prognosis (Fig. 4.1). Slow escape rates, wide QRS patterns, and fluctuating bundle branch block indicate His–Purkinje involvement or intranodal AV block. Transient failure of an escape rhythm may result in brief periods of asystole and require insertion of a temporary pacemaker (see Case 4.2). Temporary pacemakers were used in 29 of 105 cases of Lyme carditis in the United States and Europe (6).

CASE 4.1

In August, a 15-year-old athletic boy presents to the emergency department with symptoms of dizziness and shortness of breath. He had experienced generalized fatigue, myalgias, and fever for the past 3 days. He denies any history of skin rash, sore throat, or upper respiratory tract infections. He has no known previous history of heart disease.

On physical examination, his temperature is normal, his pulse rate is regular at 40 beats/min, and his blood pressure is 110/60 mm Hg. The remainder of his examination is unremarkable. Electrocardiography shows complete AV block with an escape rhythm of 42/min; the QRS configuration is normal. The chest radiograph and echocardiogram are also normal. Serologic testing for Lyme disease reveals a positive IgM antibody titer.

Prognosis

In most patients, AV block is self limited and complete recovery occurs within 6 weeks, even without antibiotic therapy (2,4). Resolution of heart block is typically gradual and progresses from complete heart block to Wenckebach and finally first-degree heart block before a return to normal sinus rhythm, presumably related to the resolution of cardiac inflammation. Persistence of conduction abnormalities lasting months after resolution of more severe block and permanent heart block have been reported but are rare. Fatalities caused by Lyme carditis have also occurred (11,12).

Myocarditis

More diffuse cardiac involvement may also occur in Lyme disease. Evidence of myocarditis includes T wave flattening or inversion, intraventricular conduction defects, ventricular premature contractions, transient and reversible depression of left ventricular function, cardiomegaly, flow murmurs, mitral regurgitation murmurs, and pericardial effusions (13).

Chest roentgenograms or echocardiograms may show cardiomegaly or an effusion (Fig. 4.2). Severe cardiac dysfunction or fulminant heart failure is rare. Pericardial effusions are typically small and not life threatening, although one case of fatal cardiac tamponade occurring in a patient with Lyme carditis has been reported (14).

Histopathologic Examinations and Immune Response

Studies of endomyocardial biopsy specimens have demonstrated the presence of infiltrates of lymphocytes and monocytes (5,8,15–17). Endocardial regions

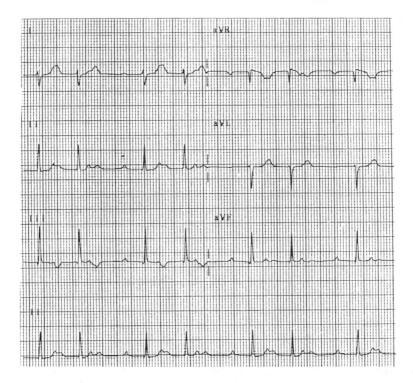

Figure 4.1   Electrocardiogram of Mobitz type 1 second-degree heart block in Lyme disease. The degree of atrioventricular block may change rapidly in patients with Lyme carditis. The majority of patients will recover completely even without antibiotic therapy. (Reprinted with permission from Evans J, Malawista S. Lyme disease. In: Mandell GL, ed. Atlas of Infectious Diseases. Vol. VIII. Philadelphia: Current Medicine; 1997:6.7.)

frequently have dense, bandlike areas of plasma cells and lymphocytes. Occasionally focal infiltrates around muscle fibers and blood vessels are found, but myocyte necrosis is unusual. Serum creatine phosphokinase (CPK) levels are typically normal. Spirochetes compatible with *B. burgdorferi* have been found near lymphoid cells and in the endocardium. The discrepancy seen at the histopathologic examination between the small number of spirochetes found and the extent of the lymphoplasmacytic infiltrate suggests that a combined effect of local spirochetal infection with an intense immunologic reaction to the organisms is responsible for disease expression.

Results from histopathologic studies carried out in mice infected with *B. burgdorferi* parallel many of the findings in human endomyocardial biopsy specimens. Sequential biopsy specimens of infected mice reveal early spirochete invasion of the heart followed by an increase in the number of spirochetes (18). Spirochetes have a predilection for connective tissue and are found near the aorta, epicardium, myocardial interstitium, and endocardium. These events coincide with periods of the most intense inflammatory response.

CASE 4.2

In July, a previously healthy 42-year-old woman is admitted to the hospital after developing fatigue on exertion. She had symptoms of dizziness and fatigue for the past 3 days. On physical examination she is pale with a normal temperature. She has an erythematous skin lesion on her back measuring 6 cm in diameter. Her pulse rate is 50 beats/min. An electrocardiogram shows complete heart block with an escape rhythm of 48 beats/min. QRS configuration is predominantly with a left bundle branch block pattern indicating a ventricular escape rhythm. The atrial rate is approximately 120/min. After admission, the patient is placed on a cardiac monitor and treatment with IV ceftriaxone is begun. The next day her heart rate drops to approximately 30 beats/min for short periods and she experiences dizziness. A temporary pacemaker is inserted. After 5 days, her heart rate increases and the complete atrioventricular block changes to a 2:1 second-degree block. Her serologic tests for Lyme disease are positive. Seven days after admission, she has first-degree heart block and is asymptomatic. She is discharged and completes a 2-week course of IV antibiotics. At 6-month follow-up, she is well, with no residual signs or symptoms of heart disease.

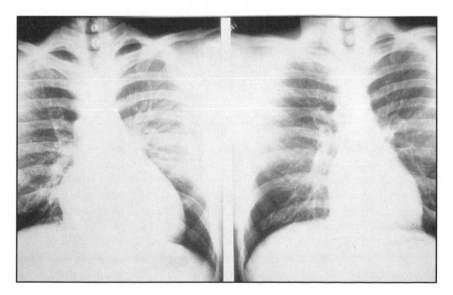

Figure 4.2   Serial chest radiographs of a patient with Lyme carditis. The heart on the left side is enlarged and suggests myocardial involvement. The radiograph on the right was taken after antibiotic therapy, and the heart has returned to normal.

In early stages, macrophages are the predominant cell type infiltrating cardiac tissue (19). Analysis of cytokine production suggests that early Lyme carditis is a direct response of macrophages to cardiac tissue invasion by *B. burgdorferi* and does not require either class II antigen expression or presentation of antigen to T-helper lymphocytes. The inflammatory response subsides as the spirochetes diminish in number. It is likely that a similar sequence of events occurs in human infection.

Chronic Cardiac Lesions

Chronic cardiomyopathy associated with Lyme disease has been reported in Europe. In 1991, *B. burgdorferi* was isolated from a patient with established dilated cardiomyopathy (17). Subsequent serologic studies in patients with chronic heart failure demonstrated a significantly higher prevalence of anti–*B. burgdorferi* antibodies in patients with dilated cardiomyopathy than in control groups (20,21).

The response to treatment with antibiotics varied. In one study, 9 patients with evidence of exposure to *B. burgdorferi* were identified from a series of 42 patients with dilated cardiomyopathy (22). All 9 received treatment with ceftriaxone, complete recovery was observed in 6 patients 6 months after therapy, and an additional 2 patients experienced partial improvement.

A second study found evidence of chronic spirochetal infection in 20 of a series of 72 consecutive patients with dilated cardiomyopathy (23). No important changes in left ventricular ejection fraction were observed to occur after antibiotic therapy. Only 2 patients, who had disease of less than 6 months' duration, showed definite clinical improvement; 1 experienced complete recovery, the other had improvement in left ventricular ejection fraction from 28% to 38% (23).

In the United States, a series of 175 consecutive patients with chronic severe heart failure were evaluated to determine the possible role of *B. burgdorferi* as an etiologic agent in chronic severe heart failure (24). No difference in overall seroreactivity between patients from endemic and nonendemic states and no correlation between serologic status and the cause of heart failure was seen. Only 2 of 13 seropositive patients had confirmatory Western blots. None of the 6 seroreactive patients who received treatment with antibiotic therapy had clinically significant improvement in left ventricular ejection fraction, indicating that Lyme disease is not a common cause of idiopathic heart failure in the United States. Similar findings were reported in the United Kingdom (25). Routine serologic screening of patients with idiopathic cardiomyopathy or aggressive antibiotic treatment for seropositive patients is not recommended unless a specific clinical history suggests antecedent Lyme disease.

Diagnosis

Lyme carditis should be considered in patients presenting with unexplained conduction disturbances and a history of exposure to *Ixodes* ticks. One should also carefully search for other clinical manifestations of Lyme disease. Nonspecific "flu-like" symptoms may have preceded the onset of cardiac disease in some patients and gone unrecognized.

Serologic confirmation of Lyme disease can usually be achieved by serologic testing in patients with Lyme carditis, although some patients may seroconvert after developing conduction disturbances. Elevation of the IgM component reflects early infection and is found in most patients with carditis. In patients with onset of carditis after 8 weeks or who have had previous exposure to Lyme disease, the level of IgG anti-*Borrelia* antibodies may be elevated. Serologic confirmation distinguishes Lyme carditis from other infections that have cardiac manifestations, such as coxsackievirus A and B, Echovirus 6 and 8, hepatitis B, *Yersinia enterocolitica*, Rocky Mountain spotted fever, and acute rheumatic fever (Box 4.2). Although myocarditis is common in Rocky Mountain spotted fever and infection with *Yersinia enterocolitica*, complete heart block is unusual. Complete heart block may occur in acute rheumatic fever but is uncommon without associated valvular involvement and congestive heart failure. In contrast, Lyme carditis is not known to involve the cardiac valves. Noninfectious causes of AV block include coronary artery disease, intracardiac operation, medication-induced AV block, congenital heart disease, idiopathic sclerodegenerative disease, fibrocalcarious encroachment, amyloidosis, sarcoidosis, and myxedema.

Abnormal gallium scans, anti-myosin-indium scans, and nuclear magnetic resonance scans have been reported in Lyme carditis but are nonspe-

---

Box 4.2   Differential Diagnosis of Lyme Carditis

Acute rheumatic fever
Other infectious diseases
  Coxsackievirus A and B
  Echovirus
  Yersinia enterocolitica
  Rocky Mountain spotted fever
Medications
  Beta-blockers
  Calcium channel blockers
  Digoxin
Coronary atherosclerotic disease
Structural cardiac abnormalities

cific (26–31). Increased gallium activity has been associated with bacterial and viral myocarditis, amyloidosis, sarcoidosis, and idiopathic congestive cardiomyopathy. In most cases of Lyme carditis, these tests are unnecessary.

Treatment and Prognosis

The optimal treatment for Lyme carditis is unknown, and to date, no studies have been performed focusing specifically on treatment of carditis. In the original clinical description of Lyme carditis, 12 of 20 patients did not receive antibiotics and received treatment with either prednisone or aspirin (2). All patients experienced complete resolution of carditis, indicating that spontaneous resolution is the rule.

Endomyocardial biopsy specimens have shown spirochete-like organisms in cardiac tissue, suggesting that direct invasion of *Borrelia* during systemic dissemination is reponsible for cardiac lesions. Although there is no evidence to suggest that antibiotics hasten the resolution of cardiac features, it is clearly prudent to treat carditis with antibiotics to eradicate systemic disease (Box 4.3).

Antibiotic Therapy

Several oral and intravenous (IV) antibiotic regimens have been successful in treating patients with Lyme carditis and preventing late sequelae of disease. Thirty-day courses of oral antibiotics such as amoxicillin, 500 mg orally three to four times per day, or doxycycline, 100 mg orally two times per day, are likely sufficient to treat milder forms of cardiac involvement such as first-degree heart block with PR intervals less than 0.3 sec.

Hospitalization with cardiac monitoring is indicated for patients with first-degree heart block with longer PR intervals, higher-degree heart block, or evidence of global ventricular impairment. Intravenous antibiotics such as penicillin G, 20 million U per day in divided doses for 14 to 28 days, and ceftriaxone, 1 to 2 g per day for 2 to 4 weeks, are recommended for such patients. Insertion of a temporary pacemaker should be considered in patients with severe and symptomatic heart block, although permanent pacing is rarely indicated.

Adjuvant Corticosteroids/Salicylates

The benefit of concomitant use of aspirin or prednisone and antibiotics in treating patients with Lyme carditis is uncertain. No clinical trials of corticosteroid or salicylate therapy versus placebo for cardiac involvement have been performed. Despite the generally benign course of Lyme carditis, several cases of permanent heart block have been reported. Concern about

---

Box 4.3   Recommendations for Management of Lyme Carditis

1. Lyme carditis should be considered in persons living or traveling in endemic areas who present with heart block, especially during the summer and fall months.
2. Patients with PR intervals ≥.03 sec should be hospitalized and placed on a cardiac monitor, because they are at the highest risk for progression to complete heart block.
3. Temporary pacemakers should be considered in patients with severe/symptomatic heart block.
4. IV ceftriaxone, 1–2 g/d for 2–4 weeks, is recommended for patients with high-degree heart block or evidence of global ventricular impairment.
5. In milder forms of heart block, 30-day courses of oral antibiotics such as amoxicillin, 500 mg orally three to four times per day, and doxycycline, 100 mg orally twice per day are sufficient.
6. Routine serologic screening of patients with idiopathic cardiomyopathy or aggressive antibiotic treatment of seropositive patients is not recommended unless a specific clinical history suggests antecedent untreated or undertreated Lyme disease.

---

potential permanent damage caused by a vigorous inflammatory response is raised when recovery is delayed.

Short courses of prednisone may be considered in patients with prolonged dense heart block to speed recovery and reduce the risk of permanent conduction system defects.

Prognosis

Recovery from Lyme carditis is generally complete without residual abnormalities or conduction disturbances within several weeks of treatment (32). Improvement from high-degree heart block typically occurs within several days of therapy, but first-degree heart block may persist longer. There are no reports of relapse of carditis occurring after therapy.

Treatment of Dilated Cardiomyopathy

Therapy for patients with dilated cardiomyopathy is uncertain. In patients with dilated cardiomyopathy and an epidemiologic profile indicating risk for infection with *B. burgdorferi,* a careful evaluation for other features of Lyme disease and serologic testing should be performed. A trial of antibiotic therapy should be considered for those patients in whom other causes of cardiomyopathy have been ruled out and with histopathologic findings consistent with Lyme carditis. Further studies are needed to determine causality and response to antibiotic treatment.

Conclusion

Lyme carditis remains a significant complication of Lyme disease. It may present quite dramatically, especially in persons who lack definitive symptoms of Lyme disease and who therefore do not receive early treatment. Complete resolution occurs in most cases, although many patients require intensive care unit monitoring and some need insertion of a temporary pacemaker. Thus far, there have been few reports of long-term cardiac sequelae after antibiotic treatment. Further studies are needed to delineate the role of Lyme disease in the pathogenesis of idiopathic cardiomyopathy.

■ ■ ■

Key Points

- Approximately 4% to 10% of patients with Lyme disease who do not receive treatment develop carditis.

- Cardiac involvement typically occurs 3 to 5 weeks after onset of infection, during the acute disseminated phase of the illness.

- Varying degrees of AV block are the most common cardiac manifestation, although myopericarditis, tachyarrhythmias, and cardiac muscle dysfunction may also be present.

- Most patients with Lyme carditis experience complete recovery, even without antibiotic therapy.

- Hospitalization, cardiac monitoring, and intravenous ceftriaxone are recommended for cases of high-degree heart block. Oral antibiotic therapy is sufficient for first-degree heart block.

■ ■ ■

REFERENCES

1. **Rubin A, Sorbera C, Nikitin P, et al.** Prospective evaluation of heart block complicating early Lyme disease. Pacing Clin Electrophysiol. 1992;15:252-5.
2. **Steere AC, Batsford WP, Weinberg M, et al.** Lyme carditis: cardiac abnormalities of Lyme disease. Ann Intern Med. 1980;93:8-16.
3. **Baylac-Domengetroy F, Vieyres C, Barraine R.** Complete heart block as the sole presentation of Lyme disease. Arch Intern Med. 1991;151:1240.
4. **McAlister HF, Klementowicz PT, Andrews C, et al.** Lyme carditis: an important cause of reversible heart block. Ann Intern Med. 1989;110:339-45.
5. **van der Linde M, Crijns H, de Koning J, et al.** Range of atrioventricular conduction disturbances in Lyme borreliosis: a report of four cases and review of other published reports. Br Heart J. 1990;63:162-8.

6. **van der Linde M.** Lyme carditis: clinical characteristics of 105 cases. Scand J Infect Dis. 1991;77:81-4.

7. **van der Linde MR, Crijins MD, Lie KI.** Transient complete AV block in Lyme disease: electrophysiologic observations. Chest. 1989;96:219-21.

8. **Reznick JW, Braunstein DB, Walsh RL, et al.** Lyme carditis: electrophysiologic and histopathologic study. Am J Med. 1986;81:923-7.

9. **Rey MJ, Zimmermann M, Adamec R, et al.** Intra-hisian 2:1 atrioventricular block secondary to Lyme disease. Eur Heart J. 1991;12:1048-51.

10. **Vlay SC, Dervan JP, Elias J, et al.** Ventricular tachycardia associated with Lyme carditis. Am Heart J. 1991;121:1558-60.

11. **Marcus L, Steere A, Duray PH, et al.** Fatal pancarditis in a patient with coexistent Lyme disease and babesiosis. Ann Intern Med. 1985;103:374-6.

12. **Cary NR, Wright DJ, Cutter SJ, et al.** Fatal Lyme carditis and endodermal heterotropia of the atrioventricular node. Postgrad Med J. 1990;66:134-6.

13. **Cox J, Krajdcn M.** Cardiovascular manifestations of Lyme disease. Am Heart J. 1991;122:1449-54.

14. **Bruyn GAW, DeKoning J, Reijsoo FJ, et al.** Lyme pericarditis leading to tamponade. Br J Rheumatol. 1994;33:862-6.

15. **de Konig J, Hoogkamp-Korstanje JAA, van der Linde MR, Crijns HJGM.** Demonstration of spirochetes in cardiac biopsies of patients with Lyme disease. J Infect Dis. 1989;160:150-3.

16. **Duray P, Steere AC.** Clinical pathologic correlations of Lyme disease by stage. Ann N Y Acad Sci. 1988;539:65-79.

17. **Stanek G, Klein J, Bittner R, Glogar D.** Isolation of *Borrelia burgdorferi* from the myocardium of a patient with longstanding cardiomyopathy. N Engl J Med. 1990; 322:249-52.

18. **Armstrong AL, Barthold SW, Persing D, Beck D.** Carditis in Lyme disease susceptible and resistant strains of laboratory mice infected with *Borrelia burgdorferi*. Am J Trop Med Hyg. 1992;47:249-58.

19. **Ruderman EM, Kerr JS, Telford SR III, et al.** Early murine Lyme carditis has a macrophage predominance and is independent of major histocompatibility complex class II-CD4+ T cell interactions. J Infect Dis. 1995;171:362-70.

20. **Stanek G, Klein J, Bittner R, Glogar D.** *Borrelia burgdorferi* as an etiologic agent in chronic heart failure? Scand J Infect Dis. 1991;77:85-7.

21. **Klein J, Stanek G, Bittner R, et al.** Lyme borreliosis as a cause of myocarditis and heart muscle disease. Eur Heart J. 1991;12(Suppl D):73-5.

22. **Gasser R, Dusleag J, Reisinger E, et al.** Reversal by ceftriaxone of dilated cardiomyopathy *Borrelia burgdorferi* infection. Lancet. 1992;339:1174-5.

23. **Bergler-Klein J, Glogar D, Stanek G.** Clinical outcome of *Borrelia burgdorferi* related dilated cardiomyopathy after antibiotic treatment. Lancet. 1992;340:317-8.

24. **Sonnesyn SW, Diehl SC, Johnson RC, et al.** A prospective study of the seroprevalence of *Borrelia burgdorferi* infection in patients with severe heart failure. Am J Cardiol. 1995;76:97-100.

25. **Rees DH, Keeling PJ, McKenna WJ, Axford JS.** No evidence to implicate *Borrelia burgdorferi* in the pathogenesis of dilated cardiomyopathy in the United Kingdom. Br Heart J. 1994;71:459-61.

26. **Jacobs JC, Rosen JM, Szer IS.** Lyme myocarditis diagnosed by gallium scan. J Pediatr. 1984;105:950-2.

27. **Alpert LI, Welch P, Fisher N.** Gallium-positive Lyme disease myocarditis. Clin Nucl Med. 1985;10:617.

28. **Casans I, Villar A, Almenar V, Blanes A.** Lyme myocarditis dagnosed by indium-111-anti-myosin antibody scintigraphy. Eur J Nucl Med. 1989;15:330-1.

29. **Globits S, Bergler-Klein J, Stanek G, et al.** Magnetic resonance imaging in the diagnosis of acute Lyme carditis. Cardiology 1994;85:415-17.

30. **Veluvolu P, Balian AA, Goldsmith R, et al.** Lyme carditis: evaluation by Ga-67 and MRI. Clin Nucl Med. 1992;17:823.

31. **Veluvolu P, Kamrani F, Horton DP, et al.** Acute transient myocarditis: evaluation by gallium imaging. Clin Nucl Med. 1992;17:411-3.

32. **Evans J, Rosenfeld L, Schoen R.** Lyme carditis: a clinical update. Ann Rheum Dis. 1993;52:402-3.

KEY REFERENCES

McAlister HF, Klementowicz PT, Andrews C, et al. Lyme carditis: an important cause of reversible heart block. Ann Intern Med. 1989;110:339-45.

A report of four serologically confirmed cases of Lyme carditis and a nice review of the literature.

Reznick JW, Braunstein DB, Walsh RL, et al. Lyme carditis: electrophysiologic and histopathologic study. Am J Med. 1986;81:923-7.

An electrophysiologic study and endomyocardial biopsy were performed in a patient with Lyme carditis. The article contains a good discussion of the histopathologic findings.

Sonnesyn SW, Diehl SC, Johnson RC, et al. A prospective study of the seroprevalence of Borrelia burgdorferi infection in patients with severe heart failure. Am J Cardiol. 1995;76:97-100.

A prospective study of 175 consecutive patients with heart failure was carried out to evaluate if B. burgdorferi was an etiologic agent in patients with idiopathic cardiomyopathy in the United States. There was no difference in overall seroreactivity between patients from endemic states and those from nonendemic states, and no correlation between the serologic status and the cause of heart failure.

Stanek G, Klein J, Bittner R, Glogar D. Isolation of Borrelia burgdorferi from the myocardium of a patient with long-standing cardiomyopathy. N Engl J Med. 1990;322:249-52.

An endomyocardial biopsy specimen obtained from a European man with dilated cardiomyopathy revealed the presence of a spirochetal organism, suggesting that Lyme disease may be a cause of chronic heart disease.

Steere AC, Batsford WP, Weinberg M, et al. Lyme carditis: cardiac abnormalities of Lyme disease. Ann Intern Med. 1980;93:8-16.

The largest case series reported of patients with Lyme carditis. Most patients had fluctuating degrees of atrioventricular block; many had changes compatible with acute myopericarditis.

5

■ ■ ■

Neurologic Manifestations
of Lyme Disease

Eric L. Logigian, MD

The clinical spectrum of Lyme neuroborreliosis is broad (1). Within days to weeks after the onset of erythema migrans, the initial skin lesion that often occurs in this infection, an early and rather distinctive neurologic syndrome occurs in about 15% of untreated patients. This syndrome consists of a lymphocytic meningitis, cranial neuropathy, or radiculoneuropathy, often appearing in combination (2–9). Less commonly, transverse myelitis or encephalitis may occur. These syndromes often improve spontaneously over several months but improve faster with antibiotic therapy.

In contrast, the chronic manifestations of the disease, which usually appear months to years after the onset of infection, are less distinctive. These manifestations of the disease do not generally resolve spontaneously but do improve, at least partially, with antibiotic therapy (10–16). The most common late manifestation of Lyme disease, in our experience (17), is a chronic encephalopathy presenting as a mild to moderately severe disorder of memory and learning (15,18). Second most common is a predominantly sensory polyradiculoneuropathy that presents either as radicular pain or distal paresthesia (1,12,14,19). The rarest late manifestation of Lyme neuroborreliosis is encephalomyelitis or leukoencephalitis (10,13,15).

Table 5.1 lists the major neurologic syndromes associated with Lyme disease and categorizes them by approximate time of appearance after disease onset.

Table 5.1   Lyme Neuroborreliosis

Syndrome	Early Onset	Late Onset
Meningitis	+	
Cranial neuropathy	+	
Severe radiculoneuropathy	+	
Encephalopathy		+
Mild radiculoneuropathy		+
Encephalomyelitis		+
Encephalitis	+	
Transverse myelitis	+	+
Meningovascular stroke		+
Inflammatory myopathy	+	+

Time Course of Neuroborreliosis

Table 5.2 delineates the chronology of Lyme disease from erythema migrans to the late neurologic manifestations, as observed in a study of 23 patients (15). The early neurologic syndrome (meningitis, cranial neuropathy, or radiculoneuropathy) appeared in 8 of the 23 patients at a median of 1 month after the development of erythema migrans. A median of 6 months later, oligoarticular arthritis developed in 70% of these patients.

Chronic peripheral nervous system involvement occurred at a median of 16 months after the onset of infection, and central nervous system involvement (encephalopathy or leukoencephalitis) developed a median of 26 months after disease onset. However, the time from erythema migrans to the onset of chronic neurologic symptoms varied widely, from 1 month to 14 years. In those patients who had had symptoms for years, there was generally little progression of the disorder over time.

Early Neurologic Syndromes

The early neurologic disorders include isolated cranial neuropathy, radiculoneuropathy, meningitis or meningoencephalitis, transverse myelopathy, and even inflammatory myopathy. However, most patients with early Lyme

Table 5.2   Time Course of Lyme Neuroborreliosis

Disorder	Time to Onset (mos)		Patients
	Median	Range	n(%)
Erythema migrans	0	—	23(85)
Early neurologic involvement	1	(0.5–2)	8(30)
Oligoarticular arthritis	6	(1–57)	19(70)
Chronic PNS involvement	16	(1–156)	19(70)
Chronic CNS involvement	26	(1–168)	21(91)

PNS = peripheral nervous system; CNS = central nervous system.
Data from Logigan EL, Kaplan RF, Steere AC. Chronic neurologic manifestations of Lyme disease. N Engl J Med. 1990;323:1438–44.

neuroborreliosis present with some combination of these syndromes, with the most common being the triad of cranial neuropathy, radiculoneuropathy, and lymphocytic meningitis (see Case 5.1) (6).

Cranial Neuropathy

Any cranial nerve, alone or in combination, can be affected, but the most common cranial neuropathy is facial palsy, which occurs in approximately 50% to 60% of patients with early neuroborreliosis (2,20). Of note, in approximately one third of such patients, facial palsy is bilateral (see Case 5.2, p 93, and Fig. 5.1, p 94). This finding is an important diagnostic point, because bilateral facial palsy is seen in only a few other conditions (e.g., Guillain-Barré syndrome, human immunodeficiency virus infection, Tangier disease, and various causes of chronic meningitis). In those patients with preceding erythema migrans, the facial palsy is most often noted within 4 weeks after the appearance of the rash (20).

As in the other syndromes of early Lyme neuroborreliosis, the most useful diagnostic tests are Lyme enzyme-linked immunosorbent assay with Western blot and a cerebrospinal fluid (CSF) examination. The purpose of examining the CSF is to document the presence of lymphocytic meningitis, which may be asymptomatic, and to determine the intrathecal presence of *Borrelia burgdorferi* with antibody testing or polymerase chain reaction (PCR) techniques. In a patient with isolated Lyme cranial neuropathy, the presence or absence of a CSF pleocytosis has important therapeutic implications:

1. The pathogenesis of Lyme cranial neuropathy is not clear. There are at least two possible mechanisms: 1) direct infection of nerve

---

CASE 5.1   *Triad of cranial neuropathy, radiculoneuropathy, and lymphocytic meningitis*

A 53-year-old man from an endemic area in New York State noted initial flu-like symptoms in September. These symptoms were followed by nagging, sharp pains that prevented him from sleeping; the pains were felt first in the right side of his neck and then in both hips and in the lower trunk. Five weeks after the on-set of his flu-like symptoms, he noted that the lower right side of his abdomen protruded whenever he tried to sit up. One week later, right facial droop was noted, followed 4 days later by left facial droop.

Examination discloses a 10 × 10 cm rash in the right side of his groin that is con-sistent with resolving erythema migrans. His neck is supple. His voice is hypo-phonic, with multiple cranial neuropathies affecting the facial, palatal, and tongue muscles bilaterally. There is also evidence of an asymmetric, multifocal polyradiculopathy with muscle weakness or sensory loss in all four limbs and the trunk. Cerebrospinal fluid examination shows 29 mononuclear cells/mm^3, an ele-vated protein level of 107 mg/dL, and a normal glucose of 62 mg/dL. The serum Lyme titers are elevated with selective concentration of antibody in CSF (5).

---

or 2) parainfectious, immunologic nerve injury. At least with re-spect to facial palsy, parainfectious mechanisms may in fact be dominant because the physiologic cause of facial paralysis is of-ten due to conduction block (e.g., demyelination), as in typical idiopathic or Bell palsy (5).

2. Recovery is excellent irrespective of treatment with antibiotics (20).

Acute Radiculoneuropathy

Early Lyme radiculoneuropathy usually presents with pain in the distribu-tion of the affected nerves and nerve roots. The pain is often severe and prevents sleep. It can be sharp and jabbing or deep and penetrating in quality. Within days to weeks, neurologic deficits accrue, resulting in sen-sory loss, weakness, or hyporeflexia. The distribution of symptoms and signs may be focal (e.g., isolated thoracic radiculopathy; see Case 5.3, p 95) but is more often multifocal and asymmetric, affecting any or all of the limbs and trunk. Occasionally, a transverse myelopathy accompanies Lyme radiculoneuritis.

The differential diagnosis of Lyme radiculoneuritis includes mechanical causes of radiculopathy, such as disc or spine disease, herpes zoster (which can occasionally produce a polyradiculoneuropathy without the typical rash, a condition termed *zoster sine herpete*), cytomegalovirus (CMV) or Epstein-Barr virus (EBV) radiculopathy, neurosarcoidosis, and di-abetic radiculoneuropathy (Table 5.3, p 96).

CASE 5.2   Isolated Cranial Neuropathy

In mid-summer, a 22-year-old female lifeguard from Cape Cod developed a numb feeling over the right upper lip, followed 1 day later by right facial palsy and 2 weeks later by left facial palsy. She does not remember receiving a tick bite or having a skin rash, and she denies headache or symptoms consistent with radiculoneuritis. The findings from her neurologic examination are entirely normal, except for bilateral facial palsy without alteration of taste or hearing. The results of the CSF examination are also normal, but both her serum IgG and IgM *B. burgdorferi* titers are elevated. She is prescribed treatment with oral doxycycline, 100 mg orally twice per day for 2 weeks. Two months after completion of therapy, her facial palsies were completely resolved.

In most patients with Lyme radiculoneuritis, serologic testing and Western immunoblot are positive for Lyme disease, a lymphocytic pleocytosis and selective concentration of *B. burgdorferi* antibody in CSF are noted (21), or the results of CSF PCR are positive for *B. burgdorferi* gene segments (22). Patients with the other conditions generally do not have a good exposure history, serologic tests are not positive for Lyme disease, and often there is specific laboratory evidence for another condition (e.g., elevated serum glucose level in diabetes, typical rash or positive CSF PCR for herpes virus, or appropriate titers in serum and CSF for EBV or CMV).

The limited pathologic data available suggest that Lyme radiculoneuritis is caused by mononuclear inflammation of nerve roots (8) and peripheral nerves (9), with the brunt of the inflammatory response in the perivascular endoneurium and perineurium. Thus far, spirochetes have not been identified within the areas of inflammation, and some have argued that nerve injury in such patients may be caused by autoantibodies to components of flagellar protein that cross-react to human axons (23). Still, the prompt response of radiculoneuritis to antibiotic therapy (within a few days to 2 weeks of therapy) suggests that active infection of nerve has a primary role in this disorder.

Lyme Meningitis

Lyme meningitis is usually heralded by prominent headache or neck pain and may take a chronic or relapsing-remitting course. A high index of suspicion is often required for this diagnosis, because it may be minimally symptomatic or even asymptomatic and signs of meningismus are often absent (see Case 5.4, p 97). CSF examination almost always shows a mononuclear pleocytosis, with elevated protein and normal glucose levels. A polymorphonuclear pleocytosis can occur rarely but should otherwise suggest another diagnosis. A selective concentration of *B. burgdorferi* antibody

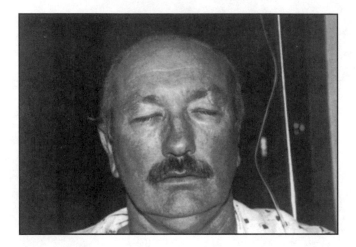

Figure 5.1   Bilateral facial palsy in Lyme cranial neuropathy. Despite trying to forcibly close his eyes, the patient could not "bury" his eyelashes. The patient also has symmetric, bilateral weakness of the lower portion of his face. (Reprinted with permission from Krishnamurthy KB, Liu GT, Logigian EL. Acute Lyme neuropathy presenting with polyradicular pain, abdominal protrusion, and cranial neuropathy. Muscle Nerve. 1993;16:1261-4.)

in CSF (usually IgG or IgA) is present in 80% to 90% of patients (23), whereas CSF PCR is positive in less than half of patients (22).

Lyme meningitis is almost certainly caused by direct infection of the meninges. In experimental infection of nonhuman primates, *B. burgdorferi* consistently gained access to the subarachnoid space 4 to 5 weeks after spirochetal inoculation of the skin (24), and in some (human) patients with acute disseminated infection, it may occur in 2 weeks or less (25). The fact that PCR testing for *B. burgdorferi* gene segments is positive in one-half or fewer patients with Lyme meningitis (22) suggests that the number of spirochetes in the CSF of these patients is very low.

Treatment of Early Lyme Neuroborreliosis

The optimal treatment regimen for early Lyme neuroborreliosis is yet to be determined. Isolated cranial neuropathy without CSF abnormalities can be treated with oral antibiotics alone, either doxycycline (100 mg orally twice per day) or amoxicillin (500 mg orally three times per day) for 2 to 4 weeks. For other manifestations of early Lyme neuroborreliosis with evidence of the spirochete in CSF, most American physicians prescribe intravenous (IV) ceftriaxone, 2 g/d for 2 to 4 weeks. We prefer to prescribe

CASE 5.3   *Isolated radiculoneuritis*

A 52-year-old female resident of Cape Cod developed "shooting" pains around her upper abdomen and inner thighs in mid-July. One week later, she noted flu-like symptoms with a fever of 101 °F (38.3 °C). The pain eventually became very severe and "penetrating" and began to prevent her from sleeping. It was not exacerbated by mechanical maneuvers. Over time, the pain became centered in the upper right quadrant.

The neurologic cause of the symptoms was not appreciated at first, and she underwent an extensive gastrointestinal evaluation, with negative findings. Eventually, the possibility of Lyme disease was raised, and a serum IgG *B. burgdorferi* titer was found to be elevated. She also had a history of a slight, daily headache and depression but no history of skin rash, stiff neck, facial palsy, or arthritis.

On examination, a thoracic sensory loss from T6-10 on the right side was noted. Other neurologic findings were normal, as were the findings of skin and joint examinations. The neck was supple, but the CSF examination showed 36 mononuclear cells/mm³ (94% lymphocytes, 2% atypical forms, 2% plasma cells); protein, 76 mg/dL; and glucose, 56 mg/dL. The CSF antibody index for *B. burgdorferi* was elevated for IgA (3.7) but normal for IgG (<1). The CSF PCR was negative.

Before our evaluation, she had received oral doxycycline, 200 mg/d for 3 weeks. We treated her with intravenous ceftriaxone, 2 g/d for 4 weeks. The pain slowly resolved after 2 weeks of therapy. At the 6-month follow-up visit, her sensory loss could no longer be demonstrated.

ceftriaxone for 4 weeks, because we have encountered patients who have had relapses or who have not completely responded to treatment after only 2 or 3 weeks of therapy. European physicians have reported satisfactory outcomes with IV penicillin, 3 g four times per day for 2 weeks, or even oral doxycycline, 200 mg/d for 2 weeks (26).

Chronic or Late Lyme Neuroborreliosis

Chronic Radiculoneuropathy

Patients with chronic radiculoneuropathy present mainly with sensory symptoms, particularly radicular pain (see Case 5.5, p 98) or distal paresthesia (see Case 5.6, p 99) in the limbs and, rarely, the trunk (11,14–16,19). Muscle weakness, if present, is slight, and there is usually no cranial neuropathy. Deep tendon reflexes are usually normal or only slightly hypoactive. Symptoms or signs can be symmetric or asymmetric, as in the radicular pain variant. Patients with distal paresthesia may present with

Table 5.3   Differential Diagnosis of Lyme Neuropathy

Acute Neuropathy	Chronic Neuropathy
Idiopathic facial palsy (Bell palsy)	Diabetes
Guillain–Barré syndrome	Other toxic–metabolic causes
Disc or spine disease	Disc or spine disease
Diabetes	Idiopathic neuropathy
Herpes zoster	Fibromyalgia
Aseptic meningitis (e.g., Epstein–Barr virus)	Leprosy
Chronic meningitis (e.g., sarcoidosis, uveomeningeal syndromes)	Perineuritis
Nonsystemic vasculitis	Wartenberg migrant neuritis

symptoms and signs in a "stocking-glove" distribution, a "stocking" distribution (see Case 5.6), or other more unusual patterns of involvement (16).

Pathogenesis

The pathology of chronic Lyme radiculoneuropathy is unknown. Because patients with this variant have symptoms similar to the well-known chronic neuropathy associated with acrodermatitis chronicum atrophicans, we assume that the pathologies of the two disorders are similar. The few nerve biopsies from patients with acrodermatitis show perivascular lymphocytic cuffing in the perineurium and endoneurium (19). To date, as with acute Lyme neuropathy (9), no spirochetes have been found in areas of nerve inflammation.

The pathogenesis of chronic Lyme neuropathy is also unknown. Because the patient's condition improves after receiving treatment with antibiotics, a role for active infection is strongly suggested. There is some evidence of an autoantibody to the flagellar protein that cross-reacts to human axons (23,27), but whether such a parainfectious immunologic mechanism for nerve injury occurs remains uncertain.

Differential Diagnosis

Table 5.4 (p 100) outlines the differences between acute and chronic Lyme radiculoneuropathy. The two are very similar, but generally the acute form is more severe and is often associated with cranial neuropathy and meningitis, whereas the chronic form is milder and may be associated with acrodermatitis. Both have a similar pathology, and in both the exact pathogenesis is unclear.

CASE 5.4   *Isolated meningitis*

A 55-year-old female resident of Cape Cod presents with a 3-month history of chronic headache that began in late summer. Findings from her physical and neurologic examinations are entirely normal, and no meningismus is present. Cerebrospinal fluid examination showed a lymphocytic pleocytosis with raised protein and normal glucose levels. Routine CSF cultures are negative. A detailed radiologic evaluation is done to exclude a parameningeal focus. The correct diagnosis is finally made when at the time of a repeat history it is learned that during mid-summer she had had a large expanding red rash on her thigh followed by severe hip pain. Her symptoms resolve after a course of intravenous penicillin.

The differential diagnosis of Lyme neuropathy, both acute and chronic, is shown in Table 5.3. For chronic neuropathy, alternative causes to consider include diabetes and compressive radiculopathy. In certain regions of the United States where chronic Lyme disease is over-diagnosed, the most common pitfall is to confuse fibromyalgia with neuropathy (17). In fibromyalgia, which does not affect nerve at all, musculoskeletal pain with multiple tender points is noted on examination, but no clear symptoms and signs of neuropathy are seen. Moreover, in contrast to Lyme neuropathy, the results of the electrophysiologic examination are normal.

Treatment
As described in Case 5.5 and Case 5.6, most patients who are treated with IV ceftriaxone for 2 to 4 weeks improve slowly, both clinically and electrophysiologically, over a period of 3 to 6 months (11,15,16,28). Because some of our patients have initially improved but subsequently relapsed after only 2 to 3 weeks of therapy, we currently recommend IV ceftriaxone for 4 weeks. We have much less experience with other antibiotic treatment regimens for this disorder.

Encephalopathy

Patients with Lyme encephalopathy generally complain of concentration and memory difficulty (12,13,15). In addition, there may be hypersomnolence, characterized by a need to take afternoon naps or go to bed early in the evening (see Case 5.7, p 101). Mild psychiatric disturbance presenting as depression, irritability, or paranoia may also develop. Patients may change their behavior to compensate for the memory disturbance, most commonly by making extensive lists to keep track of their affairs. Family members may notice that the patient forgets names of close friends or relatives and requires frequent repetition in order to learn new things. Functionally, most patients using compensatory methods can continue to work,

---

CASE 5.5   *Chronic radiculoneuropathy presenting as radicular pain*

A 53-year-old woman developed erythema migrans on her left foot in June, followed by oligoarticular arthritis affecting the left knee 7 months later, in January. Two years and three months after the onset of erythema migrans, she developed low back pain radiating into the right anterior thigh, with less pain radiating to the left thigh. She had no previous history of early Lyme neuroborreliosis, of symptoms of mechanical low back pain, or of another disease process known to produce neuropathy.

On physical examination, moderate weakness of right hip flexion and decreased vibratory sensation in her toes is noted. Electrophysiologic studies disclosed a polyradiculoneuropathy with active denervation in the L1-3 myotomes, including paraspinal muscles bilaterally, and prolonged peroneal and tibial distal motor latencies in intrinsic foot muscles. She has an elevated serum IgG Lyme titer of 1:1600, but the results of the CSF examination are normal, without pleocytosis, an elevated protein level, or a selective concentration of antibody to *B. burgdorferi*. In addition, a magnetic resonance imaging scan of the lumbosacral spine is normal.

She receives treatment with IV ceftriaxone for 2 weeks and her condition slowly improves. By 4 months after treatment, she is asymptomatic and the findings of her examination are normal.

---

but this often requires intense and constant effort. About 25% of patients have to retire or reduce their workloads.

Diagnostic Testing

The most useful tests to document Lyme encephalopathy are the CSF examination and detailed neuropsychologic tests. In more than half of the patients with this disorder, the CSF protein level is elevated or there is selective concentration of antibody to *B. burgdorferi* relative to the serum (15,21). Neuropsychologic tests usually disclose abnormalities of verbal or visual memory and sometimes mild depression (15,18). The MRI scan is abnormal in only about 25% of patients (15), with the abnormalities consisting mainly of white matter lesions, which may or may not enhance with gadolinium. More importantly, the MRI is useful to exclude other causes of encephalopathy, such as stroke, subdural hematoma, or hydrocephalus. The electroencephalogram is generally normal, or in rare cases, it may show some mild slowing. No sharp activity is seen, a finding which is consistent with the absence of seizure and myoclonus in these patients.

More recently, we have found the SPECT scan (single-photon emission computed tomography) to be useful in the diagnosis of Lyme encephalopa-

---

CASE 5.6   *Chronic radiculoneuropathy presenting as distal paresthesia*

In July, a 36-year-old woman developed erythema migrans over her chest in association with flu-like symptoms. She received appropriate treatment with doxycycline and made a rapid recovery. However, 1 month after completion of therapy, she developed "numbness and a muffled feeling," first over the medial aspect of the left great toe, then over the left foot, and then over the medial aspect of the left lower leg. No pain accompanied these symptoms.

On examination, multimodal sensory loss is noted in the distribution of the left sural, saphenous, and superficial peroneal nerves. She has normal muscle tone, power, and bulk and has normal deep tendon reflexes. Laboratory evaluation shows a sensory mononeuropathy multiplex with decreased amplitude of sensory nerve action potentials evoked from clinically affected nerves. In contrast, her distal compound muscle action potentials in intrinsic foot muscles are of normal amplitude and latencies. The results of her electromyographic examination are also normal. Her serum IgG Lyme titer is elevated at 1:400.

She receives treatment with a 2-week course of intravenous ceftriaxone, 2 g/day. By the time of her 6-month follow-up, her symptoms have resolved.

---

thy. In all of our patients with Lyme encephalopathy tested to date, the SPECT scan has shown multifocal abnormalities of perfusion, largely affecting the cerebral hemisphere white matter. It is important to note, however, that these findings are not specific for Lyme encephalopathy and can even be seen occasionally in healthy persons.

Theories of Pathogenesis

The pathology of Lyme encephalopathy is unknown, and the pathogenesis of the disorder has been debated. Some have wondered if the memory disorder is secondary to depression or chronic pain. We believe that this possibility is unlikely because patients with Lyme encephalopathy have significantly greater memory loss on neuropsychologic tests than do patients with primary depression or fibromyalgia who complain of memory difficulty (18).

Others have speculated that the cause of Lyme encephalopathy is "toxic-metabolic," stemming from coexistent systemic disease, perhaps mediated by neuromodulators diffusing from the systemic circulation across the blood–brain barrier (29). Although this mechanism is possible, systemic symptoms are usually no longer present in the patient with Lyme encephalopathy. Another possible cause is a "burnt-out" or residual leukoencephalitis following an acute encephalomyelitis. However, we believe this explanation, too, is unlikely, because most of our patients with late Lyme encephalopathy did not have early acute neuroborreliosis.

Table 5.4   Characteristics of Lyme Radiculoneuropathy

Acute Radiculoneuropathy	Chronic Radiculoneuropathy
Sensory and motor symptoms	Mainly sensory symptoms
Severe	Mild
Early onset	Later onset
Associated with cranial neuropathy and meningitis	Acrodermatitis
Improves spontaneously and with antibiotic therapy	Improves with antibiotic therapy
Perivascular infiltrate on biopsy	Perivascular infiltrate on biopsy
Pathogenesis unclear	Pathogenesis unclear

For two reasons, we favor the hypothesis that active infection of the brain is the reason for Lyme encephalopathy:

1. Many patients with this syndrome have selective concentration of antibody to *B. burgdorferi* in CSF.
2. After treatment with IV antibiotics, symptoms subjectively improve, CSF protein declines, and, on repeating testing, verbal memory and the findings on SPECT show improvement.

Given the location of SPECT scan abnormalities, it appears that active infection may particularly affect cerebral white matter, a hypothesis supported by the experimental observation that *B. burgdorferi* selectively adheres to and injures oligodendrocytes (30).

Differential Diagnosis
The differential diagnosis of Lyme encephalopathy is shown in Table 5.5, p 102. In the United States, Lyme encephalopathy is most commonly confused with chronic fatigue syndrome (17). It is also confused with depression, normal aging with slight decrease in memory, and early Alzheimer disease.

These conditions are usually easily differentiated from Lyme encephalopathy. With these other conditions, most patients do not have a good history of tick exposure or any of the early classic manifestations of Lyme disease. Indeed, we have seen only 1 in more than 100 patients with chronic neuroborreliosis who did not have early symptoms of Lyme disease, such as erythema migrans, cranial nerve palsy, radiculoneuritis, or oligoarticular arthritis. Secondly, patients with these alternative disorders usually do not have an elevated antibody response to *B. burgdorferi*.

CASE 5.7   *Chronic encephalopathy*

A 35-year-old, right-handed construction worker was well until July 1979, at which time he developed erythema migrans in association with flu-like symptoms. Four days later, right facial palsy and fatigue developed, but these resolved within 1 month. Five months later, in December, he developed oligoarticular arthritis affecting the knees, which resolved spontaneously by 1983. In 1985, 6 years after onset of infection, the patient's wife noted that he had become very forgetful and was tending to fall asleep in the afternoons while on the job. There were no symptoms of another disease process, new medicines, or drug abuse to explain his symptoms.

On examination at the bedside, the patient appeared normal. However, neuropsychologic tests showed that he had a markedly abnormal verbal memory despite a normal IQ. Cerebrospinal fluid examination showed no pleocytosis but did show an elevated protein level of 97 mg/dL. His serum Lyme titer was elevated, but more importantly, he had selective concentration of antibody to *B. burgdorferi* in CSF, with a CSF:serum ratio of 1.3. An MRI scan of the brain and a polysomnogram were normal.

He received treatment with a 4-week course of IV ceftriaxone, and his condition gradually improved over 3 to 6 months, with a decrease in his CSF protein level from 97 to 70 to 52 mg/dL. Neuropsychologic tests showed improvement but were still slightly abnormal at 6 months after therapy.

Occasionally we have seen patients with a past history of Lyme disease who have a profound memory disturbance more consistent with Alzheimer disease than with the less severe memory loss characteristic of Lyme encephalopathy. However, because of their definite early symptoms of Lyme disease, we have occasionally treated these patients for Lyme encephalopathy, but none have improved. In a recent case, the SPECT scan showed abnormalities characteristic of Alzheimer's disease rather than characteristic of Lyme encephalopathy.

Treatment
Lyme encephalopathy is treated with IV ceftriaxone, 2 g/d for 4 weeks. Improvement occurs slowly over a period of months and may not even begin until after the therapy is completed (15). Rarely, relapse has occurred after 1 month of therapy. We have treated such patients with another course of ceftriaxone for 1 month, usually with good results.

Lyme Leukoencephalitis or Encephalomyelitis

We have seen only five patients with encephalomyelitis associated with Lyme disease (see Case 5.8, p 103). Ackermann and colleagues in West

Table 5.5   Differential Diagnosis of Chronic Lyme Neuroborreliosis

Encephalopathy	Leukoencephalitis
Chronic fatigue or fibromyalgia	Multiple sclerosis
Toxic–metabolic causes	Postinfectious encephalomyelitis
Depression	
Normal aging	
Early Alzheimer's disease	
Neurosyphilis	
Other systemic inflammatory disease (e.g., lupus)	

Germany have previously reported a large series of 48 patients with this disorder (10). They described symptoms and signs of cranial neuropathy, including optic neuropathy, in association with spastic paraparesis or tetraparesis, bladder dysfunction, ataxia, dysarthria, and encephalopathy. All had a CSF pleocytosis and selective concentration of antibody to *B. burgdorferi* in CSF. They responded, at least partially, to treatment with IV penicillin.

The pathology and pathogenesis of this disorder are still unclear. As in chronic Lyme encephalopathy and radiculoneuropathy, we believe that patients with encephalomyelitis have active infection of the nervous system, because they often improve after treatment with IV ceftriaxone. Still, a parainfectious mechanism (27), triggered by infection, is also possible and may explain the large white matter lesions sometimes shown by brain MRI scans.

Lyme encephalomyelitis must be distinguished from multiple sclerosis. These two conditions are usually easy to differentiate, because patients with multiple sclerosis usually do not have a good history of tick exposure or any of the early manifestations of Lyme disease. In addition, they do not have an elevated serum Lyme titer and do not have selective concentration of antibody to *B. burgdorferi* in CSF (31).

Recommendations

Acute Lyme Neuroborreliosis

It should not be difficult to diagnose acute Lyme neuroborreliosis in patients who are residents of an endemic area and who present in the summer or fall with the triad of cranial neuropathy, radiculoneuropathy, and lymphocytic meningitis. However, it may take longer to make the correct

CASE 5.8   *Lyme leukoencephalitis*

A 39-year-old, right-handed man from Lyme, Connecticut, developed erythema migrans in June 1979. Seven months later, he noticed swelling of his right knee. In 1988, 9 years after disease onset, he began experiencing progressive gait difficulty, urinary urgency, and right-hand infacility when writing. He did not have any of the characteristic symptoms of multiple sclerosis affecting the optic nerves, the brain stem, or the dorsal columns of the spinal cord.

On examination, it is noted that he has asymmetric spasticity and weakness in the legs, increased muscle tone in the arms with slowed rapid alternating movements in the fingers, and a slow, narrow-based gait. CSF examination shows a slight pleocytosis with 8 lymphocytes/mm^3 and an elevated protein level of 67 mg/dL. Most importantly, he has selective concentration of antibody to *B. burgdorferi* in CSF, with a CSF:serum ratio of 4.0. A magnetic resonance imaging scan of the head shows periventricular white matter changes. Visual, brain stem, and somatosensory-evoked potentials are normal. He receives treatment with intravenous ceftriaxone, 2 g/d for 4 weeks, and his condition slowly improves over the next 3 to 6 months.

diagnosis unless one bears in mind that 1) patients should be questioned about travel to endemic areas; 2) some patients do not recall or develop prior erythema migrans; 3) the symptoms of meningitis may be minimal; and 4) any of the three manifestations may occur in isolation.

Patients suspected of having acute Lyme neuroborreliosis should be evaluated with serologic tests and routine CSF examination. In addition, the presence of CSF infection should be sought by obtaining paired serum and CSF samples, to exclude intrathecal production of antibody to *B. burgdorferi*, and by PCR to exclude spirochetal DNA.

Adults with CSF abnormalities should probably be treated with IV ceftriaxone 2 g/d for 2 to 4 weeks. Adults with isolated cranial neuropathy with a normal CSF examination can be treated with oral doxycycline, 100 mg twice per day, or amoxicillin, 500 mg three times per day, for 3 to 4 weeks. Improvement of symptoms of meningitis or radiculoneuritis occurs rapidly over days to weeks in early neuroborreliosis.

Chronic Lyme Neuroborreliosis

Symptoms and signs of encephalopathy, neuropathy, or encephalomyeltis are nonspecific, and most patients with these syndromes will be found to have diseases other than Lyme disease. The diagnosis of chronic Lyme neuroborreliosis is made by establishing the presence of earlier classic manifestations of Lyme disease and by testing for specific antibody. CSF samples should be obtained for routine analysis, for paired CSF and serum testing to look for selective concentration of antibody to *B. burgdorferi* in CSF, and, if available, for PCR. Neuropsychologic testing is helpful in documenting memory loss. Electrophysiologic testing often proves the presence of radiculoneuropathy. Brain MRI and SPECT scans can demonstrate white matter lesions.

The treatment with which we have the most experience is IV ceftriaxone, 2 g/d for 2 to 4 weeks. In contrast to acute Lyme neuroborreliosis, chronic neuroborreliosis shows slow improvement over many months.

■ ■ ■

Key Points

- Lyme neuroborreliosis may present as a seasonal, acute syndrome during the summer or fall or as a nonseasonal, chronic syndrome.

- The acute syndromes are distinctive and usually present as one or more of the triad: cranial neuropathy (commonly facial palsy), painful polyradiculopathy, or meningitis.

- The chronic syndromes are less distinctive and present as a mild encephalopathy, mild radiculoneuropathy, or, least commonly, encephalomyelitis.

- Because chronic syndromes are virtually always preceded by the classic early symptoms of Lyme disease (e.g., erythema migrans, cranial or radiculoneuropathy, or oligoarticular arthritis), seronegativity and the absence of the previous classic symptoms should suggest another diagnosis.

- Treatment for acute or chronic Lyme neuroborreliosis is intravenous ceftriaxone for 2 to 4 weeks; for isolated cranial neuropathy with a CSF examination with normal results, oral doxycycline or amoxicillin for 2 to 4 weeks.

■ ■ ■

REFERENCES

1. **Logigian EL, Steere AC.** Lyme borreliosis. In: Lampert HL, ed. Infections of the Central Nervous System. Philadelphia: BC Decker; 1991:218-28.
2. **Ackermann R, Horstrup P, Schmidt R.** Tick-borne meningopolyneuritis. Yale J Biol Med. 1984;57:485-90.
3. **Bannwarth A.** Zur Klinik und Pathogenese der "chronischen lymphocytaren Meningitis." Arch Psychiatr Nervenkr. 1944;117:161-85.

4. **Garin C, Bujadoux C.** Paralysie par les tiques. J Med Lyon. 1922;7:765-7.

5. **Krishnamurthy KB, Liu GT, Logigian EL.** Acute Lyme neuropathy presenting with polyradicular pain, abdominal protrusion, and cranial neuropathy. Muscle Nerve. 1993;16:1261-4.

6. **Pachner AR, Steere AC.** The triad of neurologic manifestations of Lyme disease: meningitis, cranial neuritis, and radiculoneuritis. Neurology. 1985;35:47-53.

7. **Reik L, Steere AC, Bartenhagen NH, et al.** Neurologic abnormalities of Lyme disease. Medicine. 1979;58:281-94.

8. **Schaltenbrand G.** Chronische aseptische meningitis. Nervenarzt. 1949;20:433-42.

9. **Vallat JM, Hugon J, Lubeau M, et al.** Tick-bite meningoradiculoneuritis: clinical, electrophysiologic, and histologic findings in 10 cases. Neurology. 1987;37:749-53.

10. **Ackermann R, Rehse-Kupper B, Gollmer E, Schmidt R.** Chronic neurologic manifestations of erythema migrans borreliosis. Ann N Y Acad Sci. 1988;539:16-23.

11. **Halperin JJ, Little BW, Coyle PK, Dattwyler RJ.** Lyme disease: cause of a treatable peripheral neuropathy. Neurology. 1987;37:1700-6.

12. **Halperin JJ, Luft BJ, Anand AK, et al.** Lyme neuroborreliosis: central nervous system manifestations. Neurology. 1989;39:753-9.

13. **Halperin JJ, Volkman DJ, Wu P.** Central nervous system abnormalities in Lyme neuroborreliosis. Neurology. 1991;41:1571-82.

14. **Hopf HC.** Peripheral neuropathy in acrodermatitis chronica atrophicans (Herxheimer). J Neurol Neurosurg Psychiatry. 1975;38:452-8.

15. **Logigian EL, Kaplan RF, Steere AC.** Chronic neurologic manifestations of Lyme disease. N Engl J Med. 1990;323:1438-4.

16. **Logigian EL, Steere AC.** Clinical and electrophysiologic findings in chronic neuropathy of Lyme disease. Neurology. 1992;42:303-11.

17. **Steere AC, Taylor E, McHugh GL, Logigian EL.** The overdiagnosis of Lyme disease. JAMA. 1993;269:1812-6.

18. **Kaplan RF, Meadows ME, Vincent LC, et al.** Memory impairment and depression in patients with Lyme encephalopathy: comparison with fibromyalgia and nonpsychotically depressed patients. Neurology. 1992;42:1263-7.

19. **Kristoferitsch W, Sluga E, Graf M, et al.** Neuropathy associated with acrodermatitis chronica atrophicans. Ann N Y Acad Sci. 1988;539:35-45.

20. **Clark JR, Carlson RD, Sasaki CT, et al.** Facial paralysis in Lyme disease. Laryngoscope. 1985;95:1341-5.

21. **Steere AC, Berardi VP, Weeks KE, et al.** Evaluation of the intrathecal antibody response to *Borrelia burgdorferi* as a diagnostic test for Lyme neuroborreliosis. J Infect Dis. 1990;161:1203-9.

22. **Pachner AR, Delaney E.** The polymerase chain reaction (PCR) in the diagnosis of Lyme neuroborreliosis. Ann Neurol. 1993;34:544-50.

23. **Sigal LH, Tatum AH.** Lyme disease patients' serum contains IgM antibodies to *Borrelia burgdorferi* that cross-react with neuronal antigens. Neurology. 1988; 38:1439-42.

24. **Pachner AR, Delaney E, O'Neil DVM, Major E.** Inoculation of non-human primates with the N40 strain of *Borrelia burgdorferi* leads to a model of Lyme neuroborreliosis faithful to the human disease. Neurology. 1995;45:165-72.

25. **Luft BJ, Steinman CR, Neimark HC, et al.** Invasion of the central nervous system by *Borrelia burgdorferi* in acute disseminated infection. JAMA. 1992;267:1364-7.

26. **Karlsson M, Hammers-Berggren S, Lindquist L, et al.** Comparison of intravenous penicillin G and oral doxycycline for treatment of Lyme neuroborreliosis. Neurology. 1994;44:1203-7.

27. **Aberer E, Brunner C, Sucharek G, et al.** Molecular mimicry and Lyme borreliosis: a shared antigenic determinant between *Borrelia burgdorferi* and human tissue. Ann Neurol. 1989;26:732-7.

28. **Dattwyler RJ, Halperin JJ, Volkman DJ, Luft BJ.** Treatment of late Lyme borreliosis—randomised comparison of ceftriaxone and penicillin. Lancet. 1988;1:1191-3.

29. **Halperin JJ, Heyes MP.** Neuroactive kynurenines in Lyme borreliosis. Neurology. 1992;42:43-50.

30. **Garcia-Monco JC, Fernandez Villar B, Szczepanski A, Benach JL.** Cytotoxicity of *Borrelia burgdorferi* for cultured rat glial cells. J Infect Dis. 1991;163:1362-6.

31. **Coyle PK.** Borrelia burgdorferi antibodies in multiple sclerosis patients. Neurology. 1989;39:760-1.

KEY REFERENCES

Ackermann R, Horstrup P, Schmidt R. Tick-borne meningopolyneuritis. Yale J Biol Med. 1984;57:485-90.

The largest series of patients with acute Lyme neuroborreliosis to date, with description of neurologic findings (cranial or radiculoneuropathy), and CSF analysis.

Dattwyler RJ, Halperin JJ, Volkman DJ, Luft BJ. Treatment of late Lyme borreliosis—randomized comparison of ceftriaxone and penicillin. Lancet. 1988;1:1191-3.

The only study to date (published in full form) that compares IV penicillin with IV ceftriaxone for treatment of chronic Lyme encephalopathy and neuropathy. Outcome was better with IV ceftriaxone than with IV penicillin.

Halperin JJ, Volkman DJ, Wu P. Central nervous system abnormalities in Lyme neuroborreliosis. Neurology. 1991;41:1571-82.

A large series of patients demonstrating the spectrum of CNS Lyme neuroborreliosis—meningitis, encephalomyelitis, encephalopathy—and the utility of intrathecal antibody production to demonstrate CNS infection.

Logigian EL, Kaplan RF, Steere AC. Chronic neurologic manifestations of Lyme disease. N Engl J Med. 1990;323:1438-44.

This study details the clinical and laboratory features of chronic Lyme encephalopathy, neuropathy, and leukoencephalitis, including the chronology of the various manifestations of Lyme disease from erythema migrans to chronic neurologic manifestations.

Luft BJ, Steinman CR, Neimark HC, et al. Invasion of the central nervous system by *B. burgdorferi* in acute disseminated infection. JAMA. 1992;267:1364-7.

A prospective study which demonstrates seeding of the CSF by B. burgdorferi *in two thirds of patients with acute disseminated infection of less than 2 weeks' duration.*

6

■ ■ ■

Musculoskeletal Features
of Lyme Disease

Allen C. Steere, MD

Musculoskeletal involvement, particularly arthritis, is known to be a prominent feature of Lyme disease, especially in the United States. Early in the illness, patients may experience migratory musculoskeletal pain in joints, bursae, tendons, muscle, or bone in one or a few locations at a time, frequently lasting only hours or days in a given location (1). Weeks to months later, after the development of a marked cellular and humoral immune response to the spirochete, patients who have not received treatment may have intermittent or chronic monoarticular or oligoarticular arthritis primarily in large joints, especially the knee, over a period of several years.

The diagnosis of Lyme arthritis is usually based on this characteristic clinical picture, exposure in an endemic area, and a positive IgG antibody response to *Borrelia burgdorferi* determined by enzyme-linked immunosorbent assay (ELISA) and Western blotting (2). In addition, spirochetal DNA can often be detected in joint fluid by polymerase chain reaction (PCR) (3,4). Lyme arthritis can usually be treated successfully with oral or intravenous antibiotics (5–7), but patients with certain genetic and immune markers may have persistent arthritis despite treatment with oral and intravenous antibiotics (7).

CLINICAL PICTURE

Natural History in Untreated Patients

The severity of untreated Lyme arthritis ranges from subjective joint pain, to intermittent attacks of joint swelling, to chronic synovitis. During the late

1970s, before the role of antibiotic therapy in Lyme disease was known, 55 patients with erythema migrans were studied prospectively to determine the natural history of the subsequent arthritis (1). The patients ranged in age from 2 to 59 years (mean, 26 years); 29 were male and 26 were female.

Of the 55 patients, 11 (20%) had no later manifestations of Lyme disease (1). Ten patients (18%) subsequently had brief, intermittent episodes of joint, periarticular, or musculoskeletal pain in one or a few joints at a time with long intervening periods of remission, but they never developed objective joint abnormalities. After a period of weeks to months, 28 patients (51%) had one episode or multiple intermittent attacks of frank arthritis. Most patients developed large knee effusions during the illness, but other large or small joints, the temporomandibular joint, or periarticular sites were sometimes affected (Table 6.1). Knees were generally very swollen and warm, but not particularly painful (Fig. 6.1/Plate 6). A few patients developed Baker's cysts that ruptured early. Attacks of joint swelling or periarticular pain were often brief, lasting only weeks. In most cases,

Table 6.1   Joints and Periarticular Sites Affected in Patients with Lyme Arthritis (n=28)

Site Affected	n	Site Affected	n
Joints		Periarticular sites	
Knee	27	Tendons	
Shoulder	14	Back	9
Ankle	12	Neck	6
Elbow	11	Bicipital	4
Temporomandibular	11	Lateral epicondyle	2
Wrist	10	Lateral collateral	1
Hip	9	de Quervain	1
Metacarpophalangeal	4	Bursae	
Proximal interphalangeal	4	Prepatellar	4
Distal interphalangeal	4	Subacromial	2
Metatarsophalangeal	4	Infraspinatus	2
Sternoclavicular	1	Oleocranon	2
		Sausage digits	2
		Heel pain	2

Data from Steere AC, Schoen RT, Taylor E. The clinical evolution of Lyme arthritis. Ann Intern Med. 1987;107:725-31.

only one or a few joints or periarticular sites were affected at a time (see Case 6.1). At the far end of the spectrum, the remaining 6 patients (11%) developed chronic synovitis later in the illness; of these, 2 (4%) had erosions, and 1 (2%) had permanent joint disability (1).

The number of patients who continued to have attacks of arthritis decreased by about 10% to 20% each year (1). However, attacks of joint swelling sometimes became longer in duration during the second or third year of the illness, lasting months rather than weeks. It was during this period that 10% of patients developed chronic arthritis, defined as 1 year or more of continuous joint inflammation, affecting primarily the knees. Even in this group of patients, the arthritis eventually resolved; the longest duration of continuous joint inflammation was 4 years.

Lyme Arthritis in Children

Lyme arthritis in children is similar to that in adults. However, a clinical course with arthritis as the only feature of the illness may be more common in children (see Case 6.2, p 111) (8,9). In addition, Lyme arthritis may be milder in young children than in older children or adults. Of 49 children who did not receive antibiotic therapy for Lyme arthritis, there was a direct correlation between age at onset and total duration of arthritis ($r = 0.3$, $P < 0.05$) (10). Among the youngest children (ages 2 to 4 years), the median total duration of active arthritis was only 4 weeks, whereas in teenagers (ages 13 to 15 years), the median total duration was 22 weeks. Several other forms of arthritis, such as natural and vaccine-induced rubella or parvovirus-associated arthritis, are also generally milder in young children than in adults.

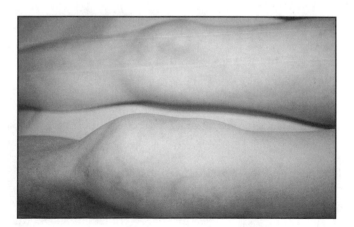

Figure 6.1   Unilateral knee effusion in Lyme arthritis. (For color reproduction, see Plate 6 at back of book.)

CASE 6.1   *Musculoskeletal pain early in the course of Lyme disease*

A 50-year-old man from Lyme, Connecticut, had a tick bite on the upper right thigh in late May. Three weeks later, he developed an enlarging, circular red rash at the site of the bite, followed by fever, arthralgias, and myalgias. Ten days later, he began to have migratory musculoskeletal pain in one or a few sites at a time, affecting the thighs and upper arms as well as the knees, shoulders, and several proximal interphalangeal joints. On physical examination, it was noted that he had a circular red lesion, 5 × 9 cm in diameter, on the right thigh; shotty inguinal lymph nodes bilaterally; a painful arc on full range of motion of the right shoulder; and tenderness on palpation of the right subacromial bursa. The ELISA test for IgM antibody to *B. burgdorferi* was positive (400 U), and the Western blot showed reactivity with the 23, 29, 41, and 58 kd spirochetal proteins, but the IgG tests were negative. He received treatment with doxycycline, 100 mg two times per day for 14 days, and had complete resolution of symptoms during the course of treatment.

In long-term follow-up, brief episodes of joint pain may sometimes occur after frank arthritis has disappeared. Of 39 untreated children with Lyme arthritis, 12 (31%) still had occasional, brief, sporadic episodes of joint pain for as long as 10 years after the period of active arthritis (10). Compared with those who became asymptomatic, the children with recurrent arthralgia more often had IgM responses to the spirochete and had significantly higher IgG titers ($P < 0.05$). Thus, in some cases, these subtle and subjective joint symptoms may have been caused by residual spirochetal infection of synovial tissue.

Lyme Arthritis in Europe

Several case series suggest that the clinical picture of Lyme arthritis is similar in the United States and Europe (11–17). However, the frequency of arthritis associated with this infection appears to be greater in the United States than in Europe. Among 55 untreated patients with erythema migrans in the northeastern United States, approximately 60% had objective evidence of arthritis (1). In contrast, in a case series of 16 untreated patients with erythema migrans in Sweden, only one (4%) developed arthritis (18). Based on these observations, it has been postulated that *B. burgdorferi* sensu stricto (19), the species that is prominent in the United States, is more arthritogenic than the European species, *Borrelia garinii* or *Borrelia afzelii* (20).

Because most patients with early infection are now treated with antibiotic therapy, the number who develop arthritis is surely less than before on both continents (21). Nevertheless, in a large epidemiologic study in Sweden carried out in 1992 and 1993, 7% of the reported cases had arthritis as a manifestation of the infection (22).

CASE 6.2   *Treatment-responsive Lyme arthritis*

A 7-year-old boy from Plymouth, Massachusetts, had a tick bite in the scalp in late June. One week later, he experienced fever for 2 days but had no other symptoms. In mid-October, 4 months later, he had the sudden onset of marked swelling in the right knee. The swelling was out of proportion to the pain. Physical examination showed a warm and swollen right knee, and shotty lymph nodes were palpable in the cervical, axillary, and inguinal chains. Sixty milliliters of joint fluid were aspirated from the knee, and the PCR test result for *B. burgdorferi* DNA in joint fluid was positive. The ELISA test for IgG antibody to *B. burgdorferi* in serum was markedly positive (25,600 U), and the Western blot showed IgG reactivity with 12 spirochetal proteins with molecular weights of 18, 23, 28, 30, 31, 34, 39, 41, 45, 58, 66, and 93 kd. He was treated with amoxicillin, 250 mg three times per day for 1 month, and had complete resolution of the arthritis during the course of treatment.

Other Musculoskeletal Manifestations

Infection with *B. burgdorferi* may occasionally cause myositis. In a series of 312 patients with early Lyme disease, 40% had myalgias, 4% had muscle tenderness on examination, and a few had severe cramping muscle pain in a localized area (23). In one case report, a patient from an area endemic for Lyme disease had fever, temporomandibular joint pain, and severe muscle pain in the left thigh and buttock (24). A gallium scan, electromyogram, and muscle biopsy suggested an inflammatory myopathy. Supporting the diagnosis of Lyme disease, the muscle biopsy showed a few spirochetes, serologic tests were positive for *B. burgdorferi*, and the patient responded to antimicrobial therapy. In a report of seven European patients with myositis as a manifestation of Lyme disease, spirochetes were found in muscle biopsies in six using silver staining (25).

Based on case reports, osteomyelitis (26) or panniculitis (27) also may occur in Lyme disease, but these reports require confirmation.

Rheumatologic Test Results

The synovial lesion in patients with Lyme arthritis is similar to that seen in other types of chronic inflammatory arthritis, including rheumatoid arthritis (28,29). Synovial biopsy specimens show synovial hypertrophy, vascular proliferation, and an infiltration of mononuclear cells, primarily lymphocytes and plasma cells, sometimes with pseudolymphoid follicles. Leukocyte counts in the joint fluid range from 500 to 110,000/μL, most of which, in patients with high leukocyte counts, are polymorphonuclear leukocytes. Tests for rheumatoid factor and antinuclear antibodies (ANA) are usually negative. However, in one study, 6 of 21 children with Lyme arthritis had positive ANAs in low titer (8).

Radiographic Findings

The most common radiographic finding is knee joint effusion (30). Intra-articular edema may be accompanied by a continuum of soft-tissue changes involving the infrapatellar fat pad, periarticular soft tissues, and the entheses, which are sometimes thickened, calcified, or ossified. Later in the illness, the joints of some patients show the typical changes of an inflammatory arthritis, including juxta-articular osteoporosis, cartilage loss, and cortical or marginal bone erosions. Less commonly, patients may exhibit changes that are more typical of a degenerative arthritis, including cartilage loss, subarticular sclerosis, or osteophytosis.

Immunogenetic Profile

Certain class II major histocompatibility genes seem to determine a host immune response to *B. burgdorferi* that results in chronic Lyme arthritis. In a study of 80 patients with Lyme arthritis, 57% of those with chronic arthritis had the HLA-DR4 specificity compared with only 23% of those with arthritis of moderate duration and only 9% of those with brief arthritis (P = 0.003) (31). In a subsequent molecular analysis of HLA class II genes in 25 patients with Lyme arthritis, 5 of the 10 patients with chronic arthritis had HLA-DR4 alleles (32). Although HLA-DR4 seems to be a risk factor for both chronic Lyme arthritis and rheumatoid arthritis, the molecular basis of the susceptibility is probably different in the two diseases.

DIAGNOSIS

Serologic Tests

The diagnosis of Lyme arthritis is usually based on the presence of a characteristic clinical picture, exposure in an area endemic for the disease, and an elevated IgG antibody response to *B. burgdorferi* (Box 6.1) (2). *Because there is a marked risk of false-positive results with serologic testing for Lyme disease, it is now recommended that all equivocal or positive results by ELISA be tested by Western blotting* (33). For the results of an IgG blot to be positive, there must be at least 5 of the 10 most common IgG bands (Box 6.1) (34). Patients with Lyme arthritis usually have high levels of IgG antibody to the spirochete with responses to many spirochetal proteins.

The limitation of serologic testing is that it does not distinguish active from inactive disease. Because patients with Lyme arthritis remain seropositive for many years after antibiotic treatment, a positive test for Lyme disease may cause diagnostic confusion if the patient subsequently develops another illness.

Box 6.1   Clues to the Diagnosis of Lyme Arthritis

- Characteristic clinical picture:
  Episodic monoarticular or oligoarticular arthritis primarily large joints, espe-
  cially the knee
- Outdoor exposure activities in an endemic area:
  Possible history of tick bite or erythema migrans
- Positive IgG antibody response to *B. burgdorferi* with reactivity with at least 5
  of the 10 most common bands: 18, 23 (OspC), 28, 30, 39, 41 (fla), 45, 58 (not
  Gro-EL), 66, 93 kd (reactivity is often found with all of these bands)
- Positive PCR test result for *B. burgdorferi* DNA in joint fluid

Polymerase Chain Reaction

Because of the limitations of serologic testing, a test is needed that identifies the spirochete itself in the joint. In most bacterial infections, culture
serves this function. However, *B. burgdorferi* has only been recovered
from joint fluid in two patients (35,36). Recently, detection of *B. burgdorferi* DNA from joint fluid by PCR has shown promise as a substitute for culture in patients with Lyme arthritis.

In a large retrospective analysis of samples obtained over a 17-year period, *B. burgdorferi* DNA was detected in 75 of 88 patients with Lyme
arthritis (85%) and in none of 64 controls (3). In this study, primer-probe
sets were used that targeted plasmid DNA encoding outer-surface protein A
(OspA) of the spirochete. In another study, synovial fluid samples from six
of seven patients with Lyme arthritis had positive PCR results using a
primer-probe set that targeted chromosomal DNA of the spirochete (4).
However, in joint fluid samples, primer-probe sets that amplify OspA plasmid DNA have generally been more sensitive than those that amplify chromosomal DNA, a phenomenon called "target imbalance" (37). To explain
this phenomenon, it has been postulated that *B. burgdorferi* in synovium
may shed OspA gene segments into joint fluid, but live spirochetes may not
always be present there.

To date, *B. burgdorferi* DNA has been detected primarily in untreated
patients with clinically active disease, suggesting that spirochetal DNA does
not persist for long after the organism has been killed. Likewise, in studies
of experimental *B. burgdorferi* infection in mice, PCR results were almost
always negative within 2 to 4 weel   after treatment with ceftriaxone (38).
Thus, a positive PCR test in synovial fluid suggests that a live spirochete is
still present within the joint.

The great problem with PCR is the risk of exogenous contamination
causing false-positive results. For this reason, PCR results must be interpreted with caution. The test is not yet routinely available.

T-Cell Proliferative Assay

In rare instances, patients may develop attenuated late manifestations of Lyme disease, including subtle joint pain or mild joint swelling, following inadequate antibiotic treatment during the first 1 or 2 weeks of early infection (39). In these patients, the humoral immune response to *B. burgdorferi* may be completely absent, but a cellular immune response can usually be demonstrated by T-cell proliferative assay.

In an initial study, 14 of 17 patients with seronegative Lyme disease had a cellular immune response to the spirochete determined by T-cell proliferative assay (39). Although other investigators have questioned the specificity of this test (40), the specificity can be improved by raising the cut-off level to 3 SD above the mean of normal controls. When this was done in a large study of 162 case-patients and controls, the sensitivity of the assay was only 45% but the specificity was 95% (41).

It should be stressed that seronegative Lyme disease is a contradiction in terms if a patient has marked arthritis, particularly chronic arthritis, because the immune response seems to be involved in the pathogenesis of joint inflammation. Seronegative Lyme disease is a subtle, attenuated illness.

Differential Diagnosis

A common problem in diagnosis is mistaking fibromyalgia or chronic fatigue syndrome for Lyme disease (Box 6.2). This problem is compounded by the fact that a small percentage of patients develop fibromyalgia in association with or soon after erythema migrans or Lyme arthritis, suggesting that *B. burgdorferi* is one of the stressful events that may trigger this chronic pain syndrome.

In a summary of the first 100 patients seen at a Lyme Disease Referral Center in New Jersey, only 37 had active Lyme disease and 25 had fibromyalgia, which was sometimes associated with Lyme disease (42). Of 788 patients evaluated at another Lyme Disease Center, 23% had active Lyme disease; 20% had previous Lyme disease and another current illness, usually chronic fatigue syndrome or fibromyalgia; and 57% did not have Lyme disease (they also most often had pain or fatigue syndromes) (43). Lyme arthritis has also been noted to be an incorrect diagnosis in pediatric or adolescent fibromyalgia (44). In a university referral center for the assessment of possible Lyme disease in British Columbia, a nonendemic area for the infection, only 2 of 65 patients were judged to have probable Lyme disease (45). Instead, 14% of the patients were diagnosed with major psychiatric illnesses and 17% with chronic fatigue syndrome or fibromyalgia.

Lyme arthritis and fibromyalgia are quite different clinically. Lyme arthritis typically causes marked joint swelling in one or a few joints at a

---

Box 6.2   Differential Diagnosis of Acute Monoarticular Arthritis

Traumatic effusion
Crystal-induced disease
Lyme arthritis
Septic arthritis
Systemic illness
   Reiter syndrome/reactive arthritis
   Juvenile rheumatoid arthritis
Erythema marginatum rheumaticum
Fibromyalgia*
Chronic fatigue syndrome

---

*Joint inflammation and lack of systemic symptoms suggest Lyme disease rather than fibromyalgia.

---

time with little in the way of systemic symptoms. This clinical picture is most like Reiter syndrome or reactive arthritis in adults or pauciarticular juvenile rheumatoid arthritis in children. In comparison, patients with fibromyalgia often have marked fatigue, headache, diffuse musculoskeletal pain, stiffness and pain in many joints, diffuse dysesthesias, difficulty with concentration, and sleep disturbance. On physical examination, such patients have multiple symmetric tender points in characteristic locations, but they lack evidence of joint inflammation (see Box 6.2).

TREATMENT

In an initial antibiotic treatment study of Lyme arthritis conducted from 1980 to 1982, 7 of 20 patients (35%) who received intramuscular benzathine penicillin, 7.2 MU, had complete resolution of joint involvement soon after treatment, compared with none of 20 patients who were given placebo ($P < 0.02$) (5). Of 20 patients treated the following year with intravenous (IV) penicillin, 20 MU/d for 10 days, 11 (55%) had complete resolution of arthritis soon after treatment. In 1983 and 1984, Eichenfield and colleagues (8) found that all 25 children with Lyme arthritis who were studied responded to treatment with either oral phenoxymethyl penicillin, 50 mg/kg per day, or tetracycline, 30 mg/kg per day, or with a combination of oral and IV antibiotics.

In 1986 and 1987, Dattwyler and colleagues (6) randomized 23 patients with Lyme arthritis, neuroborreliosis, or both to receive IV penicillin, 20 MU/d for 10 days, or IV ceftriaxone, 2 g/d for 14 days. Only 5 of the 10 patients responded to the treatment with penicillin (50%) compared with

12 of the 13 patients (92%) who received ceftriaxone. Thus, ceftriaxone is often considered to be the drug of choice for the treatment of late Lyme disease.

It has recently been reported, however, that patients with Lyme arthritis can usually be treated successfully with oral antibiotics. In a randomized study of 40 patients, 18 of 20 patients treated with doxycycline, 100 mg twice per day for 30 days, and 16 of 18 patients who completed treatment with amoxicillin plus probenecid, 500 mg of each four times per day for 30 days, had resolution of the arthritis within 1 to 3 months after entering the study (7). The major disadvantage of this approach was that neuroborreliosis developed later in 5 patients, 4 of whom had received the amoxicillin regimen. However, in retrospect, all 5 patients with this complication told of subtle peripheral dysesthesias or memory impairment at the time of their initial treatment. Thus, *when considering oral antibiotic treatment for Lyme arthritis, the physician must be alert to the presence of subtle neurologic symptoms*, which may require IV rather than oral therapy.

Treatment-Resistant Disease

A small percentage of patients with Lyme arthritis appear not to respond to either oral or IV antibiotics (*see* Case 6.3). In a case series of 16 patients who had persistent Lyme arthritis despite previous oral antibiotics or parenteral penicillin, none had resolution of arthritis within 3 months after treatment with IV ceftriaxone, 2 g/d for 14 days (7).

A major question has been whether this treatment-resistant course results from persistence of the spirochete in sequestered sites or from immune phenomena that may continue for months or even several years after the apparent eradication of live spirochetes from the joint. Recent observations based on PCR testing are compatible with the latter hypothesis. Of 10 patients who had chronic arthritis despite multiple courses of antibiotic therapy, 7 had negative PCR test results for *B. burgdorferi* DNA in all post-treatment samples and none had a positive test result after more than 2 months of treatment with oral antibiotics or 3 weeks of treatment with IV antibiotics (3).

Certain immunogenetic and immune markers have been associated with treatment-resistant Lyme arthritis. When risk factors were compared in treatment-resistant and treatment-responsive patients, the presence of either the HLA-DR4 specificity or antibody reactivity with OspA increased the odds of nonresponse, and the presence of both of these markers was associated with the greatest risk of persistent arthritis (7). When T-cell responses were compared in nine patients with treatment-responsive or treatment-resistant Lyme arthritis, OspA was preferentially recognized by T-cell lines from patients with treatment-resistant arthritis, but was only rarely

---

CASE 6.3   *Treatment-resistant Lyme arthritis*

A 44-year-old man from Oxford, New Jersey, noted an expanding circular rash on his right calf, which lasted about 2 weeks. The rash was not painful, and he had no other signs or symptoms.

Six months later, he began to experience migratory arthralgias in the shoulders, elbows, wrists, fingers, knees, and hips, in one or several locations at a time and lasting for 1 or 2 days in any given location. Six months later, he had the onset of marked swelling in the right and then the left knee. The results of a Lyme antibody test were positive. He received treatment first with oral doxycycline, but his knees remained swollen. Despite subsequent treatment with a 10-week course of IV ceftriaxone, followed by an additional 3-month course of oral antibiotic therapy, the right knee remained swollen.

He was first seen at New England Medical Center almost 2 years after disease onset. On physical examination, evidence of rotator cuff tendinitis of the left shoulder and a moderately swollen and warm right knee were seen. The ELISA test for IgG antibody to *B. burgdorferi* was markedly elevated (12,800 U), and a Western blot showed IgG responses to 12 spirochetal proteins, including reactivity with outer-surface proteins A and B (OspA and OspB). Similarly, his joint fluid and peripheral blood mononuclear cells had marked cellular immunoreactivity with these proteins. However, the PCR test result for *B. burgdorferi* DNA in joint fluid was negative. His HLA haplotype included the HLA-DRB1*0101 allele, an allele that has the same sequence in the third hypervariable region of the DRB1 chain as HLA-DRB1*0401. With treatment with anti-inflammatory agents, the swelling of the knee gradually resolved over the next 2 years. The total duration of joint swelling, even with antibiotic treatment, was nearly 4 years.

---

recognized by T-cell lines from patients with treatment-responsive arthritis (odds ratio, 28; 95% CI, 9–87; $P < 0.005$) (46). In contrast, the T-cell lines in both groups of patients frequently recognized OspB but only occasionally recognized OspC, p39, or p93. These findings help support that OspA–specific T cells have a role in the immunopathogenesis of therapy-resistant Lyme arthritis.

Recommendations

Oral doxycycline or amoxicillin for 30 to 60 days is recommended in adult patients with Lyme arthritis who do not have concomitant neurologic involvement (Box 6.3). However, the doxycycline regimen should not be used in children 8 years old or younger or in pregnant women. In case of allergy to penicillin or doxycycline, cefuroxime axetil is a possible alternative. In those with concomitant joint and neurologic involvement, IV ceftriaxone, 2 g once per day for 30 days, is recommended. After treatment, the levels of antibody to *B. burgdorferi* decline slowly over a period of months (5,6), and antibody determinations are therefore rarely helpful in assessing the adequacy of treatment. Even an apparent increase in titer must be interpreted with caution unless the samples are tested together on the same plate.

In patients who have persistent arthritis despite treatment with a 2-month course of oral antibiotic therapy or a 1-month course of oral therapy and a 1-month course of IV therapy, PCR testing of synovial fluid, if done in a reliable laboratory, may help guide decisions about retreatment. If the results of PCR testing are negative, we treat such patients with anti-inflammatory agents. Intra-articular steroids seem to be the medical modality that is most likely to provide relief of knee swelling, but we do not continue this approach if patients still develop recurrent effusions after one or two injections. If persistent joint swelling is painful or limits function, arthroscopic synovectomy may reduce the period of joint swelling (47).

The fibromyalgia syndrome, even if triggered by infection with *B. burgdorferi*, seems not to respond to antibiotic therapy (48). There is no

---

Box 6.3   Treatment Regimens for Lyme Arthritis

Arthritis (intermittent or chronic):

Adults
   Doxycycline,* 100 mg orally twice per day for 30 to 60 d†
   Amoxicillin, 500 mg orally three times per day for 30 to 60 d
   In case of doxycycline or penicillin allergy:
      Cefuroxime axetil, 500 mg orally twice per day for 30 to 60 d
Children (age ≤8 y)
   Amoxicillin, 50 mg/kg/d orally in divided doses, but not >500 mg orally, three times per day for 30 to 60 d

Arthritis and neuroborreliosis:

Ceftriaxone, 2 g IV once per day for 30 d

Persistent arthritis after >2 mo of antibiotic treatment (with PCR test result negative)

   Nonsteroidal anti-inflammatory agents
   Intra-articular steroid injection
   Arthroscopic synovectomy

---

*Doxycycline should not be used in pregnant women.
†If patients do not respond to a 30-day course of oral therapy, some physicians prefer to give IV ceftriaxone therapy for the second month rather than oral therapy.

evidence that prolonged antibiotic therapy for many months or years is of benefit in the treatment of either Lyme arthritis or fibromyalgia. In a recent cost-effectiveness analysis, it was concluded that in patients with symptoms of nonspecific myalgia and fatigue who have positive Lyme antibody test results, the risks and costs of empirical parenteral antibiotic therapy exceed the benefits (49).

■ ■ ■

Key Points

* Musculoskeletal pain in early illness may be transient or migratory, in one or a few locations at a time.

* Later disease includes intermittent episodes of monoarticular or oligoarticular arthritis, especially of the knee and large joints.

* Approximately 60% of untreated patients develop arthritis, which progresses to chronic arthritis in 10%.

* Oral doxycycline or amoxicillin for 30 to 60 days is recommended for adults who do not have neurologic symptoms.

■ ■ ■

REFERENCES

1. **Steere AC, Schoen RT, Taylor E.** The clinical evolution of Lyme arthritis. Ann Intern Med. 1987;107:725–31.
2. **Wharton M, Chorba TL, Vogt RL, et al.** Case definitions for public health surveillance. MMWR Morb Mortal Wkly Rep. 1990;39:19–21.
3. **Nocton JJ, Dressler F, Rutledge BJ, et al.** Detection of *Borrelia burgdorferi* DNA by polymerase chain reaction in synovial fluid in Lyme arthritis. N Engl J Med. 1994;330:229–34.
4. **Bradley JF, Johnson RC, Goodman JL.** The persistence of spirochetal nucleic acids in active Lyme arthritis. Ann Intern Med. 1994;120:487–89.
5. **Steere AC, Green J, Schoen RT, et al.** Successful parenteral penicillin therapy of established Lyme arthritis. N Engl J Med. 1985;312:869–74.
6. **Dattwyler RJ, Halperin JJ, Volkman DJ, Luft BJ.** Treatment of late Lyme borreliosis: randomised comparison of ceftriaxone and penicillin. Lancet. 1988;1:1191–4.
7. **Steere AC, Levin RE, Molloy PJ, et al.** Treatment of Lyme arthritis. Arthritis Rheum. 1994;37:87–88.
8. **Eichenfield AH, Goldsmith DP, Benach JL, et al.** Childhood Lyme arthritis: experience in an endemic area. J Pediatr. 1986;109:753–8.

9. **Culp RW, Eichenfield AH, Davidson RS, et al.** Lyme arthritis in children: an orthopaedic perspective. J Bone Joint Surg [Am]. 1987;69A:96–9.

10. **Szer IS, Taylor E, Steere AC.** The long-term course of children with Lyme arthritis. N Engl J Med. 1991;325:159–63.

11. **Herzer P, Wilske B, Preac-Mursic V, et al.** Lyme arthritis: clinical features, serological, and radiographic findings of cases in Germany. Klin Wochenschr. 1986;64:206–15.

12. **Blaauw I, Nohlmans L, et al.** Lyme arthritis in the Netherlands: A nationwide survey among rheumatologists. J Rheumatol. 1991;18:1819–22.

13. **Kryger P, Hansen K, Vinterberg H, Pedersen FK.** Lyme borreliosis among Danish patients with arthritis. Scand J Rheumatol. 1990;19:77–81

14. **Huaux JP, Bigaignon G, Stadtsbaeder S, et al.** Pattern of Lyme arthritis in Europe: report of 14 cases. Ann Rheum Dis. 1988;47:164–5.

15. **Ananjeva LP, Skripnikova IA, Barskova VG, Steere AC.** Clinical and serologic features of Lyme borreliosis in Russia. J Rheum. 1995;22:689–94.

16. **Huppertz H-I, Karch H, Suschke H-J, et al.** Lyme arthritis in European children and adolescents. Arthritis Rheum. 1995;38:361–8.

17. **Bianchi G, Rovetta G, Monteforte P, et al.** Articular involvement in European patients with Lyme disease: a report of 32 Italian patients. Br J Rheumatol. 1990;29:178–80.

18. **Hovmark A, Asbrink E, Olsson I.** Joint and bone involvement in Swedish patients with *Ixodes ricinus*–borne *Borrelia* infection. Zentralbl Bakteriol Mikrobiol Hyg. 1986;A263:275–84.

19. **Baranton G, Postic D, Saint-Girons I, et al.** Delineation of *Borrelia burgdorferi* sensu stricto, *Borrelia garinii* sp. nov., and group VS461 associated with Lyme borreliosis. Int J Syst Bacteriol. 1992;42:378–83.

20. **Assous MV, Postic D, Paul G, et al.** Western blot analysis of sera from Lyme borreliosis patients according to the genomic species of the Borrelia strains used as antigens. Eur J Clin Microbiol Infect Dis. 1993;12:261–8.

21. **Asch ES, Bujak DI, Weiss M, et al.** Lyme disease: an infectious and postinfectious syndrome. J Rheumatol. 1994;21:454-61.

22. **Berglund J, Eitrem R, Ornstein K, et al.** An epidemiologic study of Lyme disease in southern Sweden. N Engl J Med. 1995;333:1319–24.

23. **Steere AC, Bartenhagen NH, Craft JE, et al.** The early clinical manifestations of Lyme disease. Ann Intern Med. 1983;99:76–82.

24. **Atlas E, Novack SN, Duray PH, Steere AC.** Lyme myositis: muscle invasion by *Borrelia burgdorferi.* Ann Intern Med. 1988;109:245–6.

25. **Muller-Felber W, Reimers CD, DeKoning J, et al.** Myositis in Lyme borreliosis: an immunohistochemical study of seven patients. J Neurol Sci. 1993;118:207–12.

26. **Jacobs JC, Stevens M, Duray PH.** Lyme disease simulating septic arthritis. JAMA. 1986;256:1138–9.

27. **Kramer N, Rickert RR, Brodkin RH, Rosenstein ED.** Septal panniculitis as a manifestation of Lyme disease. Am J Med. 1986;81:149–52.

28. **Johnston YE, Durav PH, Steere AC, et al.** Lyme arthritis spirochetes found in synovial microangiopathic lesions. Am J Pathol. 1985;118:26–34.

29. **Steere AC, Duray PH, Butcher EC.** Spirochetal antigens and lymphoid cell surface markers in Lyme synovitis: comparison with rheumatoid synovium and tonsillar lymphoid tissue. Arthritis Rheum. 1988;31:487–95.

30. **Lawson JP, Steere AC.** Lyme arthritis: radiologic findings. Radiology. 1985;154: 37–43.

31. **Steere AC, Dwyer E, Winchester R.** Association of chronic Lyme arthritis with HLA-DR4 and HLA-DR2 alleles. N Engl J Med. 1990;323:219–23.

32. **Ruberti G, Begovich AB, Steere AC, et al.** Molecular analysis of the role of HLA class II genes DRB1, DQB1, and DPB1 in susceptibility to Lyme arthritis. Hum Immunol. 1991;31:20–7.

33. Centers for Disease Control. Proceedings of the Second National Conference on Serologic Diagnosis of Lyme Disease. Washington, DC, Association of State and Territorial Public Health Laboratory Directors, 1994, pp 1–111.

34. **Dressler F, Whalen JA, Reinhardt BN, Steere AC.** Western blotting in the serodiagnosis of Lyme disease. J Infect Dis. 1993;167:392–400.

35. **Snydman DR, Schenkein DP, Berardi VP, et al.** *Borrelia burgdorferi* in joint fluid in chronic Lyme arthritis. Ann Intern Med. 1986;104:798–800.

36. **Schmidli J, Hunziker T, Moesli P, Schaad UB.** Cultivation of *Borrelia burgdorferi* from joint fluid three months after treatment of facial palsy due to Lyme borreliosis. J Infect Dis. 1988;158:905–6.

37. **Persing DH, Rutledge BJ, Rys PN, et al.** Target imbalance: disparity of *Borrelia burgdorferi* genetic material in synovial fluid from Lyme arthritis patients. J Infect Dis. 1994;169:664–8.

38. **Malawista SE, Barthold SW, Persing DH.** Fate of *B. burgdorferi* DNA in tissues of infected mice after antibiotic treatment. J Infect Dis. 1994;170:1312–6.

39. **Dattwyler RJ, Volkman DJ, Luft BJ, et al.** Seronegative Lyme disease: dissociation of the specific T- and B-lymphocyte responses to *Borrelia burgdorferi*. N Engl J Med. 1988;319:1441–6.

40. **Zoschke DC, Skemp AA, Defosse DL.** Lymphoproliferative responses to *Borrelia burgdorferi* in Lyme disease. Ann Intern Med. 1991;114:285–9.

41. **Dressler F, Yoshinari NH, Steere AC.** The T cell proliferative assay in the diagnosis of Lyme disease. Ann Intern Med. 1991;115:533–9.

42. **Sigal LH.** Summary of the first 100 patients seen at a Lyme disease referral center. Am J Med. 1990;88:577–81.

43. **Steere AC, Taylor E, McHugh GL, Logigian EL.** The overdiagnosis of Lyme disease. JAMA. 1993;269:1812–6.

44. **Sigal LH, Patella SJ.** Lyme arthritis as the incorrect diagnosis in pediatric and adolescent fibromyalgia. Pediatrics. 1992;90:523–8.

45. **Burdge DR, O'Hanlon DP.** Experience at a referral center for patients with suspected Lyme disease in an area of nonendemicity: first 65 patients. Clin Infect Dis. 1993;16:558–60.

46. **Lengl-Janssen B, Strauss AF, Steere AC, Kamradt T.** The T helper cell response in Lyme arthritis: differential recognition of *Borrelia burgdorferi* outer surface protein A in patients with treatment-resistant or treatment-responsive Lyme arthritis. J Exp Med. 1994;180:2069–78.

47. **Schoen RT, Aversa JM, Rahn DW, Steere AC.** Treatment of refractory chronic Lyme arthritis with arthroscopic synovectomy. Arthritis Rheum. 1991;34:1056–60.

48. **Dinerman H, Steere AC.** Lyme disease associated with fibromyalgia. Ann Intern Med. 1992;117:281–5.

49. **Lightfoot RW Jr, Luft BJ, Rahn DW, et al.** Empiric parenteral antibiotic treatment of patients with fibromyalgia and fatigue and a positive serologic result for Lyme disease: a cost-effectiveness analysis. Ann Intern Med. 1993;119:503–9.

KEY REFERENCES

Dressler F, Whalen JA, Reinhardt BN, Steere AC. Western blotting in the serodiagnosis of Lyme disease. J Infect Dis. 1993;167:392–400.

Criteria are given for positive serologic test results for Lyme disease by ELISA and Western blot, and examples are shown of Western blots in patients with various manifestations of Lyme disease and in control subjects.

Nocton JJ, Dressler F, Rutledge BJ, et al. Detection of *Borrelia burgdorferi* DNA by PCR in synovial fluid in Lyme arthritis. N Engl J Med. 1994;330:229–34.

PCR testing of joint fluid shows promise as a substitute for culture in patients with Lyme arthritis.

Steere AC, Levin RE, Molloy PJ, et al. Treatment of Lyme arthritis. Arthritis Rheum. 1994;37:878–88.

A randomized study of doxycycline versus amoxicillin in patients with Lyme arthritis. Nonresponders were given IV ceftriaxone.

Steere AC, Taylor E, McHugh GL, Logigian EL. The overdiagnosis of Lyme disease. JAMA. 1993;269:1812–6.

The diagnoses in 788 patients referred to a university Lyme disease clinic are detailed. The most common problem in diagnosis was to mistake Lyme disease for chronic fatigue syndrome or fibromyalgia.

Steere AC, Schoen RT, Taylor E. The clinical evolution of Lyme arthritis. Ann Intern Med. 1987;107:725–31.

The natural history of Lyme arthritis is described in 55 untreated patients with erythema migrans. Subsequent joint involvement ranged from subjective joint pain, to intermittent attacks of oligoarticular arthritis, to chronic synovitis.

7

■ ■ ■

Lyme Disease in Children

Eugene D. Shapiro, MD

lthough Lyme disease is the most common vector-borne disease in the United States, extensive publicity in the lay press as well as a very high frequency of misdiagnosis have resulted in anxiety about the illness that is out of proportion to the morbidity that it causes (1,2). This anxiety is seen among physicians as well as among patients and parents.

Lyme disease was first described in children (3), but relatively few prospective studies of either the clinical course of the disease or its long-term outcomes in children have been done since its cause was discovered and appropriate antimicrobial treatment has been identified.

Epidemiology

The incidence of Lyme disease is highest in children. In Connecticut in 1995, the reported incidence among children 5 to 10 years old was 79 per 100,000 persons per year. Because only a small proportion of cases of Lyme disease are reported, these figures are undoubtedly underestimates. In a prospective study of students who attended middle school and high school in the area of Lyme, Connecticut, the rates of symptomatic and asymptomatic infection were 10 per 1,000 persons per year and 4 per 1,000 person per year, respectively (4).

Clinical Features

The clinical features of Lyme disease in children generally are similar to those reported among adults, but there are fewer reports of long-term complications of the illness. Limited data suggest that, compared with adults, children with Lyme disease are more likely to present with fever and arthritis (5–7). Reports from Europe have suggested that children with Lyme disease commonly present with either peripheral facial nerve palsies or aseptic meningitis and are less likely to present with arthritis than with neurologic symptoms (8–10). However, there may be important differences in the clinical manifestations of Lyme disease in Europe and in the United States that are related to strain-specific differences in *Borrelia burgdorferi* (1).

Erythema Migrans

In the largest prospective study of children with Lyme disease that has been reported—a community-based study of 201 children with Lyme disease in Connecticut who were enrolled in the study from April 1992 to November 1993—the median age of the children was 7 years (11). The initial (presenting) manifestations of Lyme disease in these children are shown in Table 7.1. Erythema migrans was more likely to occur on either the head or neck in younger children and on the extremities in older children, a finding similar to those recently reported from Europe (12,13). As in studies of primarily adults (10,14), only about one third of the children with a single EM rash had a positive serologic test result for *B. burgdorferi* at the time of presentation, whereas almost 90% of the children with multiple EM were seropositive. It should be noted that more than one fourth of these children had early disseminated Lyme disease at the time that they presented to a physician.

Overall, 89% of the children with Lyme disease had EM at the time that they presented to a physician. This is higher than the proportion (approximately 67%) reported in many of the early studies of Lyme disease; however, it is consistent with another prospective study recently conducted by the Connecticut Department of Health, in which 95% of persons with newly diagnosed Lyme disease had EM (15). The discrepancy between the newer and the older studies probably can be attributed to referral bias in the earlier studies (many of the study participants were referred) and to progressive improvement in the ability of physicians to recognize EM.

Of the patients with a single EM rash, 45% had received a recognized tick bite in the preceding month, but in only about half of these children was the recognized bite at the site of the rash (which indicates that the infection was transmitted by a different, unrecognized tick). Thus, a history of tick bite should be viewed as a marker for exposure to ticks, but clini-

Table 7.1   Presenting Manifestations of Lyme Disease (n=201)

Manifestation	n (%)
Single erythema migrans	132 (66)
Multiple erythema migrans	46 (23)
Arthritis	13 (6)
Facial palsy	6 (3)
Meningitis	3 (1)
Carditis	1 (0.5)
Total	201 (100)

Data from Gerber MA, Shapiro ED, Burke GS, et al. Lyme disease in children in Southeastern Connecticut. N Engl J Med 1996;335:1270-4.

cians should be aware that Lyme disease may have been transmitted by a different tick than the one that the patient recognized.

Lyme Arthritis

In the United States, neurologic disease as a manifestation of late Lyme disease is rarely, if ever, seen in children. Late Lyme disease in children virtually always manifests as arthritis. As in adults, Lyme arthritis in children is monoarticular or pauciarticular. Most (>90%) of children with Lyme arthritis present with arthritis of the knee (7).

Clinically, the child with Lyme arthritis usually presents with a subacute effusion of the knee (see Case 7.1), although occasionally the presentation may be acute and may mimic that of septic arthritis. However, the joint of a child with Lyme arthritis rarely is as exquisitely tender as it is in a child with acute bacterial arthritis. Analysis of the joint fluid generally does not help to make the diagnosis, because the findings are nonspecific and the range of observed values is wide. For example, the leukocyte count in synovial fluid can range from fewer than 10,000 to greater than 100,000 cells/mL. On the other hand, sometimes it may be useful to document that the effusion is not primarily blood, so that trauma may be ruled out as a cause of the effusion.

Nonspecific Symptoms

Among the features of Lyme disease that have led to confusion among practitioners as well as the public are the nonspecific symptoms (e.g., headache, fatigue, and arthralgia) that frequently accompany Lyme disease.

CASE 7.1   *Typical Lyme arthritis in a child*

A 10-year-old boy developed swelling in his left knee. He previously had been well, although his parents recalled that he had fallen on that knee the week before during soccer practice (a "red herring"). He had no history of fever, tick bite, or rash. On examination, the child is found to be afebrile. There is evidence of synovitis, with an effusion in the knee joint; the knee is only moderately tender. Both an enzyme-linked immunosorbent assay (ELISA) and Western blot test for infection with *B. burgdorferi* yield strongly positive results. The child receives treatment with doxycycline for 4 weeks and has a complete and rapid recovery.

Very rarely these nonspecific symptoms persist for weeks after treatment is completed, although they resolve eventually (usually within 2 to 6 months). There is no evidence that persistence of nonspecific symptoms is an indication of inadequately treated or persistent infection.

Although patients with Lyme disease often have these nonspecific symptoms at the time that they present to a physician, objective signs of Lyme disease (e.g., EM, seventh nerve palsy, or a swollen joint) also almost always are present. Patients virtually never have nonspecific symptoms as the only manifestation of Lyme disease.

Diagnosis

The diagnosis of Lyme disease in the absence of the characteristic EM rash may be difficult, because the other clinical manifestations of Lyme disease are not specific (16). It is well documented that the sensitivity and specificity of antibody tests for Lyme disease vary substantially.

The accuracy of prepackaged commercial kits is much poorer than that of tests performed by reference laboratories, which maintain tight quality control and regularly make up the materials that are used in the test. A national study of the prepackaged commercial kits was initiated by the Association of State and Territorial Public Health Laboratory Directors in conjunction with the Centers for Disease Control and Prevention (CDC) (17). In this study, different state laboratories and the CDC used the seven "best" commercial kits (as established by preliminary testing) to determine concentrations of antibodies against *B. burgdorferi* in samples of reference sera (with known positives and negatives to which the testers were blinded). The concordance of the results produced in the same laboratory using different test kits as well as the concordance of the results from different laboratories using the same test kit were poor. The overall accuracy of these commercial test kits also was poor. The estimates of the mean sensitivities of the kits ranged from 26% to 57%. The estimates of their mean specificities ranged from 12% to 60%. The investigators concluded that with these commercial diagnostic test kits, "serologic testing for Lyme disease will result in a high rate of misdiagnosis" (17). This conclusion was consistent with numerous other reports of the poor reproducibility of most commercially available antibody tests for Lyme disease (18–20).

The use of Western blot improves the specificity of serologic testing for Lyme disease (21). Official recommendations from the Second National Conference on Serologic Diagnosis of Lyme Disease suggest that clinicians use a two-step procedure when ordering antibody tests for Lyme disease (22):

1. First, use a sensitive screening test, either an ELISA or an immunofluorescent assay (IFA).

2. If that result is positive or equivocal, Western immunoblotting is used to confirm the result. If the results of the ELISA or IFA are negative, immunoblotting is not necessary.

Of course, antibody tests are not useful for the diagnosis of early localized Lyme disease, because the results are positive for only a minority of patients with EM at a single site.

Testing in Patients with Nonspecific Symptoms

The predictive value of antibody tests (even of very accurate tests) depends greatly on the prevalence of the infection among patients who are tested (23). Unfortunately, many lay persons as well as many physicians believe erroneously that nonspecific symptoms (e.g., headache, fatigue, and arthralgia) alone may be a manifestation of Lyme disease. Parents of children with nonspecific symptoms only frequently demand that the child be tested for Lyme disease, and some physicians routinely order tests for Lyme disease for such patients (see Case 7.2).

Lyme disease is the cause of these nonspecific symptoms in very few, if any, such children. However, because the specificity of even excellent antibody tests for Lyme disease rarely exceeds 90% to 95%, a great majority of the tests in children with nonspecific symptoms (>95%) yield false-positive results. Nevertheless, an erroneous diagnosis of Lyme disease frequently is made based on the results of these tests, and these children often receive unnecessary treatment with antimicrobials.

False-Positive Results

Clinicians should realize that even when serologic tests are positive for antibodies to B. burgdorferi in a symptomatic patient, Lyme disease may not

---

CASE 7.2   *Misdiagnosis of Lyme disease in a child*

A 6-year-old boy presents with a recent history of frequent episodes of pharyngi-tis and upper respiratory infections as well as transient myalgia and arthralgia. A serologic test for Lyme disease, requested by the mother and performed at a large commercial laboratory, yields a positive result. The child is prescribed treat-ment with amoxicillin for 3 weeks. After transient improvement, the symptoms recur. When the child does not respond to a second, 1-month course of amoxi-cillin, he is referred to a specialist. The results of the physical examination are en-tirely normal. Lyme titer (both ELISA and Western blot), done at a reference laboratory, are negative. The diagnosis is frequent episodes of viral respiratory infections.

---

be the cause of that patient's symptoms. In addition to the possibility that the result may be falsely positive (a common occurrence), the patient may truly have been infected with *B. burgdorferi* previously, with the current symptoms unrelated to that previous infection. Once serum antibodies to *B. burgdorferi* develop, they may persist for many years despite adequate treatment and clinical cure of the disease (24).

In addition, a substantial proportion of people who become infected with *B. burgdorferi* never develop symptoms; therefore, in endemic areas there is a background rate of seropositivity among patients who have never had clinically apparent Lyme disease (4,25,26). When patients with previ-ous Lyme disease (whether asymptomatic and untreated or clinically appar-ent and adequately treated) develop any kind of symptoms and are tested for antibodies against *B. burgdorferi*, their symptoms may erroneously be attributed to active Lyme disease because of a positive serologic test.

Congenital Lyme Disease

There is no definite evidence that *B. burgdorferi* causes congenital disease, although the existence of such a syndrome also has not been ruled out. If it does exist, congenital Lyme disease must be extremely rare. In addition, transmission of Lyme disease through breast-feeding has not been docu-mented.

Because clinical syndromes caused by congenital infection have been recognized with other spirochetal infections such as syphilis, there has been concern about the possible transmission of *B. burgdorferi* from an in-fected pregnant woman to her fetus. Although case reports have been pub-lished in which *B. burgdorferi* has been identified from several abortuses and from a few live-born children with congenital anomalies, the placentas, abortuses, and tissues from affected children in which the spirochete was identified did not show histologic evidence of inflammation (27–29).

In addition, no consistent pattern of congenital malformations (as would be expected in a "syndrome" caused by congenital infection) has been identified. In two small longitudinal studies of pregnant women who developed Lyme disease that were conducted by the CDC (30,31) and in another study conducted in the Czech Republic (32), the occasional adverse outcomes that occurred (such as spontaneous abortion) could not be attributed to infection with *B. burgdorferi*. In addition, two serosurveys conducted in endemic areas found no difference in the prevalence of congenital malformations among the offspring of women with serum antibodies against *B. burgdorferi* and the offspring of those without such antibodies (33,34). In the most comprehensive study of Lyme disease in pregnancy, investigators prospectively studied 2000 pregnant women in Westchester County, New York (35). Although the number of exposed women was relatively small, no association was found between a mother's exposure to *B. burgdorferi* either before conception or during pregnancy and fetal death, prematurity, or congenital malformations.

To assess the prevalence of clinically significant neurologic disorders attributable to congenital infection with *B. burgdorferi*, two investigators conducted a survey of all pediatric neurologists in most Lyme-endemic areas (Connecticut, Rhode Island, Massachusetts, New York, New Jersey, Wisconsin, and Minnesota) (36). Of the 162 pediatric neurologists who responded to the survey (92%), none had seen a child with a clinically significant neurologic disorder that was attributed to congenital Lyme disease or whose mother had Lyme disease during her pregnancy.

Treatment

Recommendations for the treatment of children with Lyme disease (most of which have been extrapolated from studies of adults, since no clinical trials of treatment have been conducted among children) are similar to those for adults (Box 7.1) (37,38). Children younger than 9 years of age should not be treated with doxycycline because it may cause permanent discoloration of their teeth.

Prognosis

There is a widespread misconception that Lyme disease is difficult to treat successfully and that chronic symptoms and clinical recurrences are common. In fact, the most common reason for failure of treatment is

---

Box 7.1   Antimicrobial Treatment of Children with Lyme Disease

Early Disease

Erythema migrans and early disseminated disease
- Doxycycline,* 100 mg bid for 21 days
  or
- Amoxicillin, 50 mg/kg/d tid (maximum 500 mg/dose) for 21 days
  or for those who cannot take amoxicillin or doxycycline,
- Cefuroxime axetil, 30–50 mg/kg/d bid (maximum 500 mg/dose) for 21 days
  or
- Erythromycin, 30–50 mg/kg/d divided qid (maximum 250 mg/dose) for 21 days

Neurologic disease†
- Ceftriaxone, 50–80 mg/kg/d in a single dose (maximum 2 g) for 14–21 days, administered IV or IM
  or
- Penicillin G, 200,000–400,000 U/kg/d (maximum 20 MU/day) q4h, administered IV for 14–21 days

Late Disease

Arthritis
- Initial treatment is the same as for erythema migrans, except duration of treatment is 30 days.‡

---

*Do not use doxycycline in children <9 years old.
†Patients with cranial neuritis (e.g., facial nerve palsy) should receive treatment with an orally administered antibiotic for 3 to 4 weeks.
‡If symptoms fail to resolve after 2 months or if they recur, some experts prescribe a second course of an orally administered antibiotic; others treat as for neurologic disease.

---

misdiagnosis (i.e., the patient's symptoms are not caused by Lyme disease) (39–41). As with adults, chronic, nonspecific symptoms associated with Lyme disease may be caused by fibromyalgia (42). The common misconceptions that Lyme disease often requires very prolonged treatment (sometimes with intravenously administered antimicrobials) and that even then treatment often is unsuccessful no doubt are, in part, the result of the treatment of patients whose symptoms are not caused by Lyme disease.

Although there are few long-term follow-up studies of treated children, the prognosis for children treated for early Lyme disease is excellent. A recent review of 65 children who were treated for EM found that at follow-up a mean of more than 3 years later, all were well and none had developed symptoms of late Lyme disease (43). In a different prospective follow-up study of children with newly diagnosed Lyme disease of any stage (although most had early-localized or early-disseminated disease), all of the children were clinically cured at follow-up a median of 2.5 years later (11).

The long-term prognosis for patients who are treated for late Lyme disease also is excellent. Although recurrences of arthritis do occur rarely, especially among patients with the HLA-DR2, DR3, or DR4 haplotypes, most children who receive treatment for Lyme arthritis are permanently cured (44). Indeed, even in children with Lyme arthritis who did not receive treatment (or who received treatment years after the onset of the arthritis), the arthritis diminished over time in both frequency and severity and eventually ceased in almost all of the children (45).

Although there are rare reports of adults who have developed late neuroborreliosis after being treated for Lyme disease (in most instances, there were long delays before treatment was initiated) (46), studies of children who have received treatment indicate that the prognosis for unimpaired cognitive function is excellent (47). Indeed, one group of investigators performed neuropsychologic tests in children with Lyme disease 4 years after they were treated and found no evidence of any long-term sequelae of the infection (47,48). Other investigators who are conducting a community-based study of the long-term outcomes of Lyme disease have also found no evidence of impairment of normal functioning in children 4 to 10 years after they were diagnosed with Lyme disease (49).

Recommendations

- Children with only nonspecific symptoms, such as headache, fatigue, or arthralgia, are very unlikely to have Lyme disease. Serologic tests for Lyme disease should not be ordered for such patients, because a positive test result is very likely to be a false-positive. Because of the low risk of Lyme disease and the excellent prognosis of children who do develop Lyme disease, prophylactic antimicrobial treatment is not indicated for children who are bitten by a deer tick.

- Orally administered treatment is recommended for children with most forms of Lyme disease (except carditis and CNS infection). Children with EM should be treated with doxycycline or amoxicillin for 2 to 3 weeks (children <9 years old should not receive doxycycline). Children with early disseminated Lyme disease should receive treatment for 3 weeks; children with Lyme arthritis should receive treatment for 4 weeks.

■ ■ ■

Key Points

- The incidence of Lyme disease is highest in children.

- Nearly 90% of children who develop Lyme disease have either single or multiple sites of erythema migrans.

- Although children with Lyme disease often have nonspecific symptoms on presentation, objective signs of Lyme disease (e.g., erythema migrans, facial palsy, or swollen joint) are also almost always present.

- There is no evidence that congenital Lyme disease is a problem.

- The prognosis of children with Lyme disease, both early and late, is excellent, with no evidence of chronic symptoms or long-term sequelae.

- Because of the low risk of Lyme disease and the excellent prognosis of children who do develop Lyme disease, prophylactic antimicrobial treatment is not indicated for children who are bitten by a deer tick.

■ ■ ■

REFERENCES

1. **Steere AC.** Lyme disease. N Engl J Med. 1989;321:586-96.
2. **Aronowitz RA.** Lyme disease: the social construction of a new disease and its social consequences. Milbank Q. 1991;69:79-112.
3. **Steere AC, Malawista SE, Snydman DR, et al.** Lyme arthritis: an epidemic of oligoarticular arthritis in children and adults in three Connecticut communities. Arthritis Rheum. 1977;20:7-17.
4. **Feder HM Jr, Gerber MA, Cartter ML, et al.** Prospective assessment of Lyme disease in a school-aged population in Connecticut. J Infect Dis. 1995;171: 1371-4.
5. **Petersen LR, Sweeney AH, Checko PJ, et al.** Epidemiological and clinical features of 1,149 persons with Lyme disease identified by a laboratory-based surveillance in Connecticut. Yale J Biol Med. 1989;62:253-62.
6. **Williams CL, Strobino B, Lee A, et al.** Lyme disease in childhood: clinical and epidemiologic features of ninety cases. Pediatr Infect Dis J. 1990;9:10-4.
7. **Eichenfield AH, Goldsmith DP, Benach JL, et al.** Childhood Lyme arthritis: experience in an endemic area. J Pediatr. 1986;109:753-8.

8. **Christen HJ, Hanefeld F, Eiffert H, Thomssen R.** Epidemiology and clinical manifestations of Lyme borreliosis in childhood: a prospective multicentre study with special regard to neuroborreliosis. Acta Paediatr. 1993;386:1-75.

9. **Dressler F.** Lyme borreliosis in European children and adolescents. Clin Exp Rheumatol. 1994:12 (Suppl 10):S49-54.

10. **Berglund J, Eitrem R, Ornstein K, et al.** An epidemiologic study of Lyme disease in southern Sweden. N Engl J Med. 1995;333:1319-24.

11. **Gerber MA, Shapiro ED, Burke GS, et al.** Lyme disease in children in Southeastern Connecticut. Pediatric Lyme Disease Study Group. N Engl J Med. 1996;335: 1270-4.

12. **Christen HJ, Bartlau N, Hanefeld F, et al.** Peripheral facial palsy in childhood: Lyme borreliosis to be suspected unless proven otherwise. Acta Paediatr Scand. 1990;79:1219-24.

13. **Jorbeck HJA, Gustafsson PM, Lind HCF, Stiernstedt GT.** Tick-borne borrelia-meningitis in children. Acta Paediatr Scand. 1987;76:228-33.

14. **Aguero-Rosenfeld ME, Nowakowski J, McKenna DF, et al.** Serodiagnosis of early Lyme disease. J Clin Microbiol. 1993;31:3090-5.

15. State of Connecticut Department of Public Health. Lyme disease; Connecticut, 1994. Connecticut Epidemiologist 1995;15:13-6.

16. **Gerber MA, Shapiro ED.** Diagnosis of Lyme disease in children. J Pediatr. 1992;121:157-62.

17. Bacterial Zoonoses Branch, Centers for Disease Control. Evaluation of serologic tests for Lyme disease: Report of a national evaluation. Lyme Disease Surveillance Summary 1991; 2:1-3.

18. **Schwartz BS, Goldstein MD, Ribeiro JMC, et al.** Antibody testing in Lyme disease: a comparison of results in four laboratories. JAMA. 1989;262:3431-4.

19. **Luger SW, Krauss E.** Serologic tests for Lyme disease: interlaboratory variability. Arch Intern Med. 1990;150:761-3.

20. **Hedberg CW, Osterholm MT.** Serologic tests for antibody to *Borrelia burgdorferi*: another Pandora's box for medicine? [editorial]. Arch Intern Med. 1990; 150:732-3.

21. **Dressler F, Whalen JA, Reinhardt BN, Steere AC.** Western blotting in the serodiagnosis of Lyme disease. J Infect Dis. 1993;167:392-400.

22. Recommendations for test performance and interpretation from the Second National Conference on Serologic Diagnosis of Lyme Disease. MMWR Morb Mortal Wkly Rep. 1995;44:590.

23. **Seltzer EG, Shapiro ED.** Misdiagnosis of Lyme disease: when not to order serologic tests. Pediatr Infect Dis J. 1996;15:762-3.

24. **Feder HM Jr, Gerber MA, Luger SW, Ryan RW.** Persistence of serum antibodies to *Borrelia burgdorferi* in patients treated for Lyme disease. Clin Infect Dis. 1992;15:788-93.

25. **Steere AC, Taylor E, Wilson ML, et al.** Longitudinal assessment of the clinical and epidemiological features of Lyme disease in a defined population. J Infect Dis. 1986;154:295-300.

26. **Hanrahan JP, Benach JL, Coleman JL, et al.** Incidence and cumulative frequency of endemic Lyme disease in a community. J Infect Dis. 1984;150:489-96.

27. **Schlesinger PA, Duray PH, Burke BA, et al.** Maternal-fetal transmission of the Lyme disease spirochete, *Borrelia burgdorferi.* Ann Intern Med. 1985;103:67-8.

28. **MacDonald AB, Benach JL, Burgdorfer W.** Stillborn following maternal Lyme disease. N Y State J Med. 1987;87:615-6.

29. **Weber K, Bratzke HJ, Neubert U, et al.** *Borrelia burgdorferi* in a newborn despite oral penicillin for Lyme borreliosis during pregnancy. Pediatr Infect Dis J. 1988;7:286-9.

30. **Markowitz LE, Steere AC, Benach JL, et al.** Lyme disease during pregnancy. JAMA. 1986;255:3394-6.

31. **Ciesielski CA, Russell H, Johnson S, et al.** Prospective study of pregnancy outcome in women with Lyme disease [abstract 39]. Presented at the Twenty-Seventh International Conference of Antimicrobial Agents and Chemotherapy, New York, 1987.

32. **Hercogová J, Hulínská D, Zivny J, Janovská D.** Erythema migrans during pregnancy: study of 35 women [Abstract D648]. Presented at VII International Congress on Lyme Borreliosis, San Francisco, June 1996.

33. **Williams CL, Benach JL, Curran AS, et al.** Lyme disease during pregnancy: a cord blood serosurvey. Ann N Y Acad Sci. 1988;539:504-6.

34. **Nadal D, Hunziker UA, Bucher HU, et al.** Infants born to mothers with antibodies against *Borrelia burgdorferi* at delivery. Eur J Pediatr. 1989;148:426-7.

35. **Strobino BA, Williams CL, Abid S, et al.** Lyme disease and pregnancy outcome: a prospective study of two thousand prenatal patients. Am J Obstet Gynecol. 1993;169:367-74.

36. **Gerber MA, Zalneraitis EL.** Childhood neurologic disorders and Lyme disease during pregnancy. Pediatr Neurol. 1994;11:41-3.

37. **Rahn DW, Malawista SE.** Lyme disease: recommendations for diagnosis and treatment. Ann Intern Med. 1991;114:1472-81.

38. **Shapiro ED.** Lyme disease. In: Burg FD, Ingelfinger JR, Wald ER, Polin RA, eds. Current Pediatric Therapy. Vol 15. Philadelphia: WB Saunders; 1995: 605-7.

39. **Steere AC, Taylor E, McHugh GL, Logigian EL.** The overdiagnosis of Lyme disease. JAMA. 1993;269:1812-26.

40. **Sigal LH.** Persisting complaints attributed to chronic Lyme disease: possible mechanisms and implications for management. Am J Med. 1994;96:365-74.

41. **Feder HM Jr, Hunt MS.** Pitfalls in the diagnosis and treatment of Lyme disease in children. JAMA 1995;274:66-8.

42. **Sigal LH, Patella SJ.** Lyme arthritis as the incorrect diagnosis in pediatric and adolescent fibromyalgia. Pediatrics. 1992;90:523-8.

43. **Salazar JC, Gerber MA, Goff CW.** Long-term outcome of Lyme disease in children given early treatment. J Pediatr. 1993;122:591-3.

44. **Zemel LS, Gerber MA, Shapiro ED.** Lyme arthritis in children: clinical epidemiology and long-term outcomes [abstract 1131]. Pediatr Res. 1995;37:191A.

45. **Szer IS, Taylor E, Steere AC.** The long-term course of Lyme arthritis in children. N Engl J Med. 1991;325:159-63.

46. **Shadick NA, Phillips CA, Logigian EL, et al.** The long-term clinical outcomes of Lyme disease: a population-based retrospective cohort study. Ann Intern Med. 1994;121:560-7.

47. **Adams WV, Rose CD, Eppes SC, Klein JD.** Cognitive effects of Lyme disease in children. Pediatrics. 1994;94:185-9.

48. **Rose CD, Fawcett WV, Adams WV, et al.** Cognitive effects of Lyme disease in children: a 4-year follow-up controlled study [abstract D656]. Presented at the VII International Congress on Lyme Borreliosis, San Francisco, June 1996.

49. **Shapiro ED, Seltzer EG, Gerber MA, Cartter ML.** Long-term outcomes of children with Lyme disease [Abstract #1094]. Pediatr Res. 1996;39:185A.

KEY REFERENCES

Gerber MA, Zalneraitis EL. Childhood neurologic disorders and Lyme disease during pregnancy. Pediatr Neurol. 1994;11:41-3.

The authors surveyed all pediatric neurologists in most areas of the United States in which Lyme disease is endemic. None had seen a patient whose symptoms they could attribute to congenital Lyme disease.

Gerber MA, Shapiro ED, Burke GS, et al. Lyme disease in children in southeastern Connecticut. N Engl J Med. 1996;335:1270-4.

The only community-based, prospective, longitudinal study of Lyme disease in children in the United States. It reviews the typical clinical manifestations of Lyme disease as well as the results of laboratory tests in these children. The excellent prognosis for children with Lyme disease is demonstrated in their more than 2.5 years of follow-up.

Salazaar JC, Gerber MA, Goff CW. Long-term outcome of Lyme disease in children given early treatment. J Pediatr. 1993;122:591-3.

Illustrates the pitfalls of diagnosing Lyme solely on the basis of serologic tests. Persons with only nonspecific symptoms and a positive serologic test result most likely do not have Lyme disease.

Seltzer EG, Shapiro ED. Misdiagnosis of Lyme disease: when not to order serologic tests. Pediatr Infect Dis J. 1996;15:762-3.

Follow-up of more than 60 children who had had erythema migrans at an average of 3 years after they were diagnosed and treated showed that none had chronic or recurrent Lyme disease (although 11% had had new episodes of erythema migrans from new tick bites).

8

■ ■ ■

Long-Term Consequences
of Lyme Disease

Leonard H. Sigal, MD

Lyme disease represents organ dysfunction caused by an infection that is antibiotic-sensitive. If left untreated, the disease may progress to later features of the infection (1). Within days to months of the initial infection, early disseminated Lyme disease may occur, which may include neurologic or cardiac disease. Months to years after the onset of infection, late Lyme disease, manifesting as neurologic or articular problems, may occur. These features of early disseminated or late Lyme disease may occur in the absence of previous erythema migrans or other earlier features of Lyme disease (up to 50% of patients with Lyme disease do not recall an erythema migrans lesion (1), although a recent study of pediatric Lyme disease found that erythema migrans was present in 90% of all cases of Lyme disease (2).

Because these later medical problems may be the first manifestations of the infection, it is important to consider Lyme disease in the differential diagnosis of the appropriate clinical problems—for example, lymphocytic meningitis, heart block, or monoarthritis. *It is equally important to remember that Lyme disease is not the most common cause for these problems, even in endemic areas.*

When these or other problems occur, Lyme disease should not be diagnosed simply because there is no other readily available explanation. In other words, Lyme disease should not become a "diagnosis of exclusion" (3)—it is not "the great imitator" (4,5). Likewise, persistence of symptoms or objective problems after therapy should not immediately be assumed to represent ongoing infection.

Diagnosis and Treatment of Lyme Disease and the Question of Active Infection

Most patients with Lyme disease are cured if they receive appropriate therapy (the correct agent, dose, duration, and method of administration), especially if treatment is received early in infection (6–8). Although a very small proportion of patients have disease progression despite receiving proper therapy during early Lyme disease (1), such patients should receive treatment appropriate for the later feature of Lyme disease (6,7). In the evaluation of patients with "later features" of Lyme disease, it is crucial to ensure that the patient's symptoms are in fact caused by Lyme disease and related to active infection; all that follows an episode of Lyme disease is not necessarily Lyme disease!

Active Lyme disease (i.e., active infection with *Borrelia burgdorferi*) is associated with *objective evidence of organ damage or dysfunction and with serologic evidence of exposure to* B. burgdorferi. Isolated symptoms are not proof of active infection. Objective evidence of Lyme disease includes physical findings and abnormalities in objective testing, such as neuropsychologic testing, electrophysiologic testing, and spinal fluid or synovial fluid analysis.

However, even objective clinical findings in association with true seropositivity (defined as a positive test result with enzyme-linked immunosorbent assay [ELISA] corroborated by Western immunoblotting) may not represent active Lyme disease. A person with persistent seropositivity from a previous infection with *B. burgdorferi* may develop an objective abnormality not caused by the previous Lyme disease. For instance, a swelling in the knee that occurs a few years after an episode of Lyme disease may actually be caused by gout or meniseal damage rather than by active *B. burgdorferi* infection of the knee. Although objective findings plus serologic evidence of *B. burgdorferi* exposure is usually necessary, these findings are not sufficient for diagnosing *active B. burgdorferi* infection with absolute assurance. The seropositivity and the synovitis in this case are not caused by Lyme disease.

As noted in Chapter 10 ("Use of the Laboratory in the Confirmation and Management of Lyme Disease"), testing of inflammatory fluids can be crucial in determining if the closed-space inflammatory process is in fact caused by *B. burgdorferi*. However, the only way to *confirm* that Lyme disease is the cause is to check the synovial fluid for crystals or blood to ensure that there is remarkable concentration of specific antibodies to *B. burgdorferi* in comparison to the serum. Even if the results of this comparison are negative, the possibility of Lyme disease still exists, given the fact that no laboratory assay is perfect.

The Natural History of Treated Lyme Disease: Symptoms Occurring After Treatment of Lyme Disease

Patients with erythema migrans may have lingering nonspecific complaints, including headache, achiness, and fatigue, persisting for as long as 6 months after treatment (1). Occasionally these symptoms may begin after treatment has concluded. However, because these symptoms resolve without further treatment, there is no reason to believe that they represent persisting infection. Persistence of such symptoms may represent the slow waning of the systemic immune reaction to *Borrelia burgdorferi*, analogous to the debility that follows hepatitis or infectious mononucleosis (see Case 8.1).

Lyme carditis usually begins to clear shortly after the start of antibiotic treatment, although persistent—and rarely, permanent—first-degree atrioventricular block has been described. Meningitis caused by *B. burgdorferi* also usually resolves after the start of treatment. Both of these conditions may be self-limited and may resolve before treatment.

Seventh cranial nerve palsy usually resolves quickly, but there have been cases of slow resolution and of permanent damage. The synovitis of Lyme arthritis may persist for 6 months or longer before beginning to re-

---

CASE 8.1   *Nonspecific, self-limited complaints occurring after Lyme disease*

A 38-year-old man from Ohio first noted an asymptomatic, expanding, ring-shaped, red rash in his left popliteal fossa 4 months ago. He states that he had been picnicking in an area of New Jersey known to be "full of Lyme disease." Upon his arrival home in Ohio, he was well except for the expanding rash. After the diagnosis of Lyme disease was made by his primary care physician, he received a 3-week course of doxycycline, which he tolerated well, and the rash disappeared within the first 10 days of treatment. He now has had symptoms of headache, fatigue, and achiness "all over" for 2 to 3 months and asks if he still has Lyme disease.

Physical examination reveals no abnormalities. Serologic testing reveals a negative IgG and IgM ELISA. The erythrocyte sedimentation rate is 2 mm/h, and the complete blood count is normal.

The likelihood that the patient's symptoms are the nonspecific symptoms that sometimes occur after the treatment of Lyme disease, and do not represent active infection, is discussed, and the patient accepts this as a reasonable explanation. At follow-up 3 months later, he is well and without symptoms. His previous symptoms decreased steadily over the first 2 months after his last visit.

solve, and the synovitis may be refractory to treatment with antibiotics. Tertiary neuroborreliosis usually responds gradually, persisting for 1 year or more before substantive improvement occurs.

Subtle cognitive dysfunction or musculoskeletal pain (9–11) may rarely develop after antibiotic therapy for early localized Lyme disease.

One explanation for ongoing symptoms in patients with previous Lyme disease is the persistence of infection with *B. burgdorferi*. In most referral practices, such a phenomenon is uncommon, although it may occur (3,12,13). It is also possible that these patients had subclinical disseminated infection at the time of their treatment and that their progressive debility might thus result from the inadequacy of their previous treatment; there is a correlation between delay in treatment or less aggressive treatment and chronic neurologic dysfunction (9,10). Long-term follow-up of these patients is not available, but many clinicians prescribe treatment with intravenous (IV) antibiotics to eradicate possible persisting infection (3–12). It is crucial to perform cerebrospinal fluid analysis and neuropsychologic testing in patients with subtle cognitive dysfunction or unusual headaches to determine if central nervous system infection exists, which then would warrant further therapy. One must also consider other potential causes and not allow "chronic Lyme disease" to become a diagnosis of exclusion in such patients (see Case 8.2).

Lyme Disease as a Diagnosis of Exclusion

In patients with chronic, nonspecific symptoms and no obvious diagnosis, the diagnosis of "chronic" Lyme disease may be made all too readily (12,13). Occasionally, these symptoms start after documented Lyme disease, although more often, the previous diagnosis of Lyme disease has not been proved. Many patients with musculoskeletal pain, fatigue, or memory and concentration problems actually have fibromyalgia (12–16) (Table 8.1, p 142). The diagnosis of Lyme arthritis is often made despite an absence of joint inflammation, or the diagnosis of tertiary neuroborreliosis is based on vague or nonspecific cognitive symptoms in the absence of objective central nervous system dysfunction. In many cases, the original diagnosis of Lyme disease is very much in doubt.

Fibromyalgia is often not considered in patients with subjective symptoms of fatigue, musculoskeletal pain, and concentration or memory difficulties but with no objective findings of Lyme disease. Fibromyalgia can occur after Lyme disease (indeed, the sleep disorder and muscle deconditioning seen in Lyme disease may predispose to fibromyalgia [3]), but fibromyalgia does not respond to further antibiotic therapy (14–16). The consequences of treating all patients with fibromyalgia who happen to have an ELISA positive for Lyme disease have been described (17).

CASE 8.2 *Persistent infection with* **Borrelia burgdorferi**

A 53-year-old man from Long Island, New York was diagnosed with arthritis of the left knee approximately 1 year ago and received steroid injections several times for "inflammation." The knee is intermittently very swollen but only mildly to moderately painful. No other joints are affected.

On examination, it is noted that the left knee is red, hot to the touch, and swollen, with a diminished range of motion owing to discomfort. Aspiration reveals 85 mL of cloudy yellow fluid with a leukocyte count of 27,000 /mm³. Serum and synovial fluid analyses are both positive for anti–*B. burgdorferi* antibodies. Immunoblot of the synovial fluid reveals IgM reactivity with the 34-kd (OspB) antigen, which is not present in serum. A diagnosis of Lyme arthritis is made, and the patient receives IV ceftriaxone for 4 weeks (he requested IV rather than the recommended oral treatment).

His arthritis resolves, and he is well for 4 months, when his right knee becomes swollen, red, and hot to the touch. Aspiration reveals 75 mL of cloudy yellow fluid with a leukocyte count of 19,500 /mm³; synovial fluid and serum analyses are both positive for anti–*B. burgdorferi* antibodies, with a preferential concentration of antibodies in the synovial fluid as compared with serum. The results of the fluid Gram stain and culture are negative, and no crystals are seen. A diagnosis of Lyme arthritis, occurring after IV antibiotic therapy, is made, and he receives treatment with cefotaxime for a further 4 weeks.

Seven months later, he still has intermittent swelling of the right knee (the left knee remains asymptomatic), and an arthroscopic synovectomy is performed (he refused the offer of treatment with hydroxychloroquine). Six months later, he is well with no further swelling in either knee.

Fibromyalgia is a musculoskeletal pain syndrome that seems to be predicated on sleep disorder and muscular deconditioning. The fatigue and concentration and memory difficulties seem to be related to the sleep disorder (18,19) (see Case 8.3, p 143). Lyme disease also may be associated with a sleep disorder, which is usually self-limited but may persist (3,15). Patients whose condition is misdiagnosed as chronic Lyme disease may also have medical conditions other than fibromyalgia, including brain tumors, rheumatoid arthritis, anti-cardiolipin antibody syndrome, and multiple sclerosis (12–16).

The persisting biologic and psychologic effects of previous infection with *B. burgdorferi* may include sleep disorder, inactivity and muscle disuse, depression, and anxiety. The cognitive dysfunction that occurs with depression, fibromyalgia, anxiety, or primary sleep disorder can mimic the cognitive dysfunction of late Lyme disease (3,9). Formalized neuropsychologic testing can be of great use in such circumstances. Although the pattern of abnormality seen in patients with Lyme disease is not unique, it is

Table 8.1   Lyme Disease Contrasted with Fibromyalgia

Characteristic	Lyme Disease	Fibromyalgia
Musculoskeletal	Evidence of inflammatory joint disease: warmth, swelling, redness, stiffness	Achiness not limited to joints: minimal or absent morning stiffness or stiffening after prolonged inactivity
		No true arthritis; no objective evidence of Lyme cardiac or neurologic disorders
Neurologic	Fatigue often associated with objective findings of disease	Evidence of primary sleep disorder: difficulty falling or staying asleep; awakening in the morning unrefreshed
	Neurocognitive abnormalities in a pattern suggestive of Lyme disease	Cognitive changes may suggest anxiety, depression, hypervigilance (which is not the pattern of Lyme disease)
Responsiveness to antibiotics	Response to treatment with antibiotics, although may be delayed	No response to treatment with antibiotics; possible good response to aerobic exercise and sleep restitution, although may be delayed

sufficiently different from the patterns that occur with depression, anxiety, head trauma, or Alzheimer's disease to differentiate Lyme disease from many other causes of concentration and memory deterioration.

A Framework for Determining the Cause of Persisting Symptoms

Given the frequency of persisting symptoms and the concern in certain populations about "chronic" Lyme disease, we need to formulate plausible explanations for "Lyme disease" that persists despite previous therapy (3). The three pivotal questions to answer are:

1. What is the pathogenesis of Lyme disease?

CASE 8.3   *Fibromyalgia misdiagnosed as "chronic" Lyme disease*

A 36-year-old female bank vice president presents for the evaluation of "chronic" Lyme disease. Approximately 7 months ago, she went to see a "Lyme disease expert" concerning her symptoms of concentration and memory problems, profound fatigue necessitating afternoon naps, and total body aches. He told her that she had "late-stage central nervous system Lyme disease" and needed intensive treatment. She received IV ceftriaxone for 6 weeks, followed by IV vancomycin and azithromycin for 8 weeks, followed by 16 weeks of trimethoprim/sulfamethoxazole plus clarithromycin alternating weekly with azithromycin and ciprofloxacin. With each regimen, she felt somewhat better, only to feel the return of her symptoms within 7 to 10 days after discontinuation of treatment. She presents to her physician concerned that she may never have had Lyme disease.

She describes a frenetic work schedule that has prevented her from taking any free time off for the last 3 years, which in fact led to a divorce about 8 months ago. Her treating physician identified a "flu-like illness" three summers ago as the start of her Lyme disease and did a "blood test for Lyme disease" that was read as being positive: an IgM of 1.2 and an IgG of 0.91 on ELISA (normal, <0.8; equivocal, 0.8 to 1.2; positive, >1.2). IgM immunoblot revealed reactivity with the 41- and 23-kd bands and IgG reactivity with the 58-kd band.

She describes awakening in the morning feeling "as if she hadn't slept at all." She describes achiness not localized to joints, intermittent crampy abdominal pain, occasional loose stools, and severe headaches often on awakening.

Examination reveals no evidence of inflammatory joint disease and a normal neurologic evaluation. Multiple tender points fulfilling the criteria for the diagnosis of fibromyalgia are noted. She is prescribed nortriptyline for sleep, aerobic exercise, and discontinuation of further antibiotics. She returns 6 weeks later feeling "better, but not back to normal." With further exercise and continuation of medication to maintain normal sleep patterns, she improves progressively and discontinues the nortriptyline after about 1 year. She continues to feel very achy after viral syndromes or during times of exceptional stress.

---

   2. What are the presumed mechanisms for symptoms that occur after antibiotic treatment (both adequate and inadequate)?

   3. How are these proposed mechanisms expected to respond to antibiotic therapy?

The Pathogenesis of Lyme Disease

B. burgdorferi is inoculated into the skin by the bite of an infected tick. Because the organism does not produce toxins or cause direct tissue damage, it is presumed that the inflammatory response to the organism causes the erythema migrans. Early dissemination of the organism to other sites occurs, with the heart and neurologic systems the most commonly affected.

In early Lyme disease, *B. burgdorferi* is identified by histochemical or immunohistochemical staining, its DNA amplified by polymerase chain reaction (PCR), or the organism cultured from cardiac and brain tissue specimens and spinal fluid samples of patients with disease affecting those organs. The organism has never been identified in or isolated from affected peripheral nerve. In late Lyme disease, *B. burgdorferi* can be grown in culture or its DNA identified by PCR from synovial fluid and brain biopsy specimens of patients with Lyme arthritis and tertiary neuroborreliosis, respectively.

Thus, evidence suggests that the organism is at the site of inflammation (with the exception of the neuropathy of early disseminated disease). The combination of the paucity of this organism at any site of disease plus sampling error may explain the absence of the organism in peripheral nerves; alternatively, the pathogenesis of neuropathy may not depend on local infection (3).

Proposed Mechanisms for Persisting Symptoms That Occur After Antibiotic Therapy

Active Infection

With active infection, *B. burgdorferi* persists alive at the site of disease. This raises the question: Why did the organism survive despite what should have been adequate therapy?

Previous therapy may have been inadequate. The dose may have been too low, the duration may have been too short, or the treatment may have been inappropriate (incorrect drug or route of administration). (For example, consider a patient with erythema migrans and severe headache, who actually has an evolving meningitis and who is prescribed treatment with an oral agent for 14 days; the duration and route of administration are likely inadequate for the features of disease.) The agent may have been absorbed poorly, or the patient may not have taken the drug properly. There has been no report of a *B. burgdorferi* isolate resistant to antimicrobials in current usage. Thus, having survived the initial therapy, over time the organisms increase in number or migrate to sites of later disease, resulting in ongoing or persisting infection.

If persisting infection is suspected, the clinician must search for objective evidence of disease: evidence of *B. burgdorferi* or the immune response to the organism in blood samples and at the site of disease, demonstrable physical findings, objective cognitive testing—and *not* isolated subjective complaints. Patients with persisting infection usually respond to appropriate antibiotic therapy. Most patients with "chronic" Lyme disease who do not respond to this therapy do not have ongoing infection with *B. burgdorferi.*

It has been claimed that the organism hides within cells or becomes "dormant" and therefore is not sensitive to antibiotics. Survival of *B. burgdorferi* within cultured murine macrophage-like cell lines in vitro suggests that the organism may evade macrophage killing once it has been ingested in vivo (20). *B. burgdorferi* has been described as entering cultured human fibroblasts and survives intracellularly in vitro, as well (21). Through such evasion of the immune system and antibiotics, the organism may survive to cause later disease, although there is no proof that this in vitro phenomenon occurs in vivo.

It is difficult, and perhaps incorrect, to extrapolate from in vitro cultures to the internal milieu of a patient. Predicating clinical practice on such an extrapolation is highly questionable, at best. There are case reports of the persistence of the organism within ligamentous tissue (22), the heart (23), and skin (24), the latter in a patient previously treated with antibiotics. However, these reports give examples of the rare exception rather than the rule. No studies to date have documented that the organism regularly becomes "dormant."

In the overwhelming majority of patients, Lyme disease resolves as the outcome of antibiotic treatment. The possibility of rare lack of response to therapy is not a cogent argument in favor of long-term therapy, given our current understanding of Lyme disease.

Patients with "chronic" Lyme disease may report a response of their symptoms within days of starting antibiotics, only to have them return within days of stopping treatment. Given the long doubling-time of *B. burgdorferi,* it is unlikely that such a rapid return of symptoms is due to a reaccumulation of a borrelial biomass sufficient to cause recrudescence of disease.

Equally at odds with what is known about the biology of this organism are the reports of a "Jarisch-Herxheimer reaction" with each treatment; the reaction can occur within a few days of the initiation of treatment (1) but is not an ongoing feature of disease. Such reports should raise doubts about the veracity of the diagnosis of Lyme disease.

Persistence of Dead Organism as a Target of the Immune System

The dead organism may persist as effete hulk or debris resistant to degradation. If the organism is dead but its antigens persist, they could remain as a focus of inflammation (25). In vitro studies have shown that *B. burgdorferi* can elicit cytokine production by human mononuclear cells—for example, interleukin-1 (26) and interleukin-6 (27). If these cytokines were produced within the synovial cavity or neuraxis, they might cause local tissue dysfunction and damage or local immune dysregulation. Activation of T-helper cells by these antigens might drive local immune reactivity (28).

The antigen-induced arthritis model, which depends on the intra-articular persistence of a foreign antigen as the focus of inflammation, may help in understanding persisting synovitis of Lyme disease. Gondolf and colleagues (29) used a butanol extract of *B. burgdorferi* to induce an antigen-induced arthritis model. Persistence of outer-surface protein A (OspA) and other borrelial components within the inflamed rat knee served as the inducing antigen and the local focus of persisting inflammation.

It is possible that perivascular persistence of borrelial antigens and subsequent local inflammation may explain the vasculopathy seen (25). In biopsies from a few patients with Lyme neuropathy, mild vasculopathy was identified in peripheral nerve (30), although no spirochetal forms were identified. A lesion suggestive of endarteritis obliterans has been identified in the inflamed synovial tissue of some patients with Lyme arthritis (31).

Thus, there are several plausible explanations for ongoing symptoms with objective evidence of tissue dysfunction or inflammation not caused by active infection. Without live organisms, further antibiotic therapy offers no benefit other than a placebo effect or possible nonantimicrobial effects (32).

It may be very difficult to differentiate between active infection and the mechanisms described above. In rare cases, serologic testing may be useful—for example, a significant increase in positive ELISA results corroborated by an expansion of the immunologic repertoire demonstrated by Western blot may be used to determine active, ongoing infection. If the patient does not respond to what should be adequate antibiotic therapy (or to ongoing or repeated therapies), this can be considered evidence that active infection is *not* the cause of the symptoms.

Persistence of the Clinical Disease After the Organism Has Been Entirely Eliminated

Damage caused during infection may evolve slowly, as damaged tissue dies or scars, so that clinically apparent tissue damage that occurs during infection may not improve after treatment. Organ damage may be clinically silent or manifest as minimal dysfunction during infection and emerge later. Such a process is postulated in the "post-polio syndrome" now becoming increasingly common in those who survived poliomyelitis in the 1950s.

A single study suggests that *B. burgdorferi* may trigger a postinfectious reactive arthritis that is analogous to Reiter syndrome (33). If a component of a microorganism resembles a component of the host, the immune response to the microbe might recognize the host component and damage the host; this is known as *molecular mimicry* (34). We have previously found cross-reactivity between *B. burgdorferi* flagellin and a human axonal protein (35), now known to be chaperonin-HSP60, a heat shock protein (36). A single monoclonal anti-flagellin antibody modifies the growth of neural cells in vitro (37), although the in vivo relevance of these findings is not yet known.

Other Disease as Cause of the Symptoms

Intercurrent illness *can* occur, and it therefore should not be assumed that all medical problems occurring after Lyme disease are necessarily caused by previous Lyme disease. One can have Lyme disease, be cured, and then develop another illness; one can also be improperly diagnosed initially.

It is only by disabusing the patient of the incorrect diagnosis that proper management can begin. This can be difficult, because many patients are convinced of the fact of their Lyme disease, having read extensively in the literature of the "alternative counterculture" (38) that has developed about Lyme disease.

Two other infectious diseases are known to occur after the bite of ixodid ticks: infections with *Babesia microti* (babesiosis) and *Ehrlichia* species (human granulocytic ehrlichiosis) (Table 8.2). Babesiosis manifests with fever, hemolytic anemia, and severe constitutional symptoms (39,40). Patients can be co-infected with *B. burgdorferi* and *B. microti,* and approximately 20% of patients with babesiosis have clinical and serologic evidence of concurrent Lyme disease (41). Human granulocytic ehrlichiosis can cause fever, headache, and constitutional symptoms, as well (39,42).

Patients with especially severe constitutional symptoms in early Lyme disease may possibly be co-infected with one of these two infections. Alternatively, some patients may have a misdiagnosis of Lyme disease and a missed diagnosis of babesiosis or ehrlichiosis. Babesiosis is treated with clindamycin and quinine, whereas ehrlichiosis responds to treatment with tetracyclines.

Conclusion

It is crucial that the diagnosis of Lyme disease be made on the basis of a history of plausible exposure to the disease, objective clinical findings suggesting organ damage or dysfunction, and (usually) serologic evidence of exposure to the etiologic agent. A diagnosis based on less than these parameters may be incorrect. Lack of response to antibiotic therapy should not be considered evidence that "chronic" Lyme disease is the explanation for the patient's current symptoms. In patients with previous, even well-documented Lyme disease, a thorough differential diagnosis is mandatory: The current symptoms should not be ascribed to Lyme disease as a diagnosis of exclusion. Recrudescence of symptoms shortly after the termination of adequate antibiotic treatment is uncommon in Lyme disease and should suggest that the underlying problem was either not an infection or that the infectious organism was not *B. burgdorferi.* Symptoms that occur after treatment for Lyme disease may occur as a result of the natural history of the response of this infection, the evolution of permanent damage caused by Lyme disease, side effects of antibiotics, or other diseases unrelated to *B. burgdorferi.*

Table 8.2   Comparison of Tick-Borne Disease: Lyme Disease, Babesiosis, and Human Granulocytic Ehrlichiosis

Borrelia burgdorferi *Infection*	Babesia microti *Infection*	Ehrlichia sp. *Infection*
Low-grade fever	High fevers possible	High fevers possible
	Constitutional symptoms predominate, can be severe	Constitutional symptoms predominate, can be severe
Erythema migrans (single or multiple)	Erythema migrans absent unless there is co-infection with *B. burgdorferi*	Erythema migrans absent unless there is co-infection with *B. burgdorferi*
Cardiac and/or neurologic features possible early	Thrombocytopenia and/or hemolytic anemia	
Minimal leukocytosis and no cytopenia		
Serologic confirmation in most patients if disease duration >4–6 wk	Serologic tests for Lyme disease negative (unless there is co-infection)	Serologic tests for Lyme disease negative (unless there is co-infection)
	Specific serologic tests for anti–*B. microti* antibodies may be positive	Specific serologic tests for anti–*B. microti* antibodies may be positive
	Thick smear of peripheral blood may reveal intra-erythrocytic parasites	Peripheral blood smear may reveal inclusion bodies within granulocytes (morulae)
Response (usually) to treatment with amoxicillin or doxycycline	Lack of response to amoxicillin or doxycycline	Lack of response to amoxicillin but response to tetracyclines

It may be useful to divide the problems related to Lyme disease into three related entities: Lyme borreliosis, post–Lyme disease syndromes, and Lyme anxiety.

Lyme Borreliosis

Lyme borreliosis consists of the features of active infection. Other less clearly established features include ophthalmopathy, chronic congestive cardiomyopathy, and other neurologic problems not within the defined syndrome.

Post–Lyme Disease Syndromes

Post-Lyme disease syndromes can be diagnosed when there is evidence of previous infection that has been adequately treated with antibiotics and there is no evidence of current active infection. In this category are fibromyalgia (caused by chronic sleep disorder and muscle deconditioning) and patellofemoral joint dysfunction (caused by inactivity or knee arthritis–related quadriceps femoris atrophy).

Studies suggest that the host immune response may cause immune-mediated damage, with proposed examples including reactive arthritis and autoimmune neuropathy. Rarely, evidence of vasculopathy has been found in biopsy specimens and may be caused by ongoing inflammation to persisting antigen in or near vessel walls. The antigen-induced arthritis model may be of relevance in understanding persisting synovitis, especially the intermittent flares of arthritis seen in late Lyme disease.

Lyme Anxiety

Lyme anxiety is common in and near areas endemic for Lyme disease. There is widespread concern that Lyme disease is incurable and that this infection can only be brought into temporary remission and will continue to flare. With widespread anxiety about Lyme disease has come Munchausen syndrome and Munchausen syndrome-by-proxy in those concerned about "chronic" Lyme disease. The psychologic and financial costs of the misdiagnosis and treatment of "chronic" Lyme disease are staggering but have not been considered in most discussions of the public health burden of the mismanagement of Lyme disease (43).

In some of the patients with "Lyme anxiety," no objective evidence of inflammation or infection is found, preceding or current, and serologic evidence of prior exposure to *B. burgdorferi* may or may not be present. Quite often, a low-positive ELISA result is the only such evidence, raising concerns of false-positive serologic testing. Not infrequently such patients have sought the advice of support groups or local "Lyme disease experts."

This category of illness represents an enlarging majority of the "chronic Lyme disease" population. Such patients have often been tested repeatedly, often with tests of no value (e.g., urinary antigen tests), and have been subjected to many courses of antibiotics, often with agents of no proven efficacy. Many patients have found a place in their personas for "chronic Lyme disease," and this may be the most permanently damaging aspect of Lyme disease.

In response to anxiety about Lyme disease has come a trend toward antibiotic regimens of greater duration or dose and combinations of antibiotics. However, this increased exposure to antibiotics results in a greater risk of adverse reactions to therapy (32,44). Not infrequently, drug side effects have been misinterpreted as manifestations of Lyme disease and occasionally labeled as "delayed Herxheimer reactions." Diarrhea in the setting of chronic antibiotic therapy has been called "Lyme colitis," an entity that has never been described in the peer-reviewed medical literature, rather than *Clostridium difficile* enteropathy; several patients with this condition have responded well to vancomycin therapy, prompting some clinicians to claim that vancomycin is a cure for borrelial enteropathy. With the emergence of enterococcus and perhaps *Staphylococcus aureus* resistant to vancomycin, the unnecessary use of this agent is to be avoided. Especially in patients receiving long-term antibiotic therapy, further antibiotic treatment is not warranted. A detailed evaluation to ensure that no other illness is present is needed, with special attention to possible fibromyalgia. Such patients need reassurance and education, not medication, to feel comfortable with their new understanding that they do not have Lyme disease.

■ ■ ■

Key Points

- Active, ongoing infection is *not* the most common cause for persisting symptoms in patients with Lyme disease who have received adequate previous antibiotic therapy.

- Before diagnosing Lyme disease, chronic or otherwise, the physician must seek objective evidence of infection; diagnosis should not be predicated on isolated symptoms, even if the patient is seroreactive.

- Screening serologic tests for Lyme disease, in the absence of symptoms, are not useful. A diagnosis should never be made on the basis of isolated serologic reactivity.

- Other diseases occurring after treatment for Lyme disease (e.g., fibromyalgia) and the side effects of antibiotics for treatment are sometimes mistaken for "active" or "chronic" Lyme disease.

■ ■ ■

REFERENCES

1. **Steere AC.** Lyme disease. N Engl J Med. 1989;321:586-96.
2. **Gerber MA, Shapiro ED, Burke GS, et al.** Lyme disease in children in southeastern Connecticut. N Engl J Med. 1996;335:1270-4.

3. **Sigal LH.** Persisting complaints attributed to chronic Lyme disease: possible mechanisms and implications for management. Am J Med. 1994;96:365-74.

4. **Pachner AR.** *Borrelia burgdorferi* in the nervous system: the new "great imitator." Ann N Y Acad Sci. 1988;539:56-64.

5. **Finkel MJ, Halperin JJ.** Nervous system Lyme borreliosis: revisited. Arch Neurol. 1992;49:102-7.

6. **Sigal LH.** Current drug therapy recommendations for the treatment of Lyme disease. Drugs 1992;43:683-99.

7. **Rahn DW, Malawista SE.** Lyme disease: recommendations for diagnosis and treatment. Ann Intern Med. 1991;114:472-81.

8. **Magid DJ, Schwartz BS, Craft J, Schwartz JS.** Prevention of Lyme disease after tick bite: a cost-effectiveness analysis. N Engl J Med. 1992;327:534-42.

9. **Logigian EL, Kaplan RF, Steere AC.** Chronic neurologic manifestations of Lyme disease. 1990;323:1438-44.

10. **Shadick NA, Phillips CB, Logigian EL, et al.** The long-term clinical outcomes of Lyme disease: a population-based retrospective cohort study. Ann Intern Med. 1994;121:560-7.

11. **Asch ES, Bujak DI, Weiss M, et al.** Lyme disease: an infectious and postinfectious syndrome. J Rheumatol. 1994;21:454-61.

12. **Sigal LH.** Summary of the first one hundred patients seen at a Lyme disease referral center. Am J Med. 1990;88:577-81.

13. **Steere AC, Taylor E, McHugh GL, Logigian EL.** The overdiagnosis of Lyme disease. JAMA. 1993;269:1812-6.

14. **Sigal LH, Patella SJ.** Lyme arthritis as the incorrect diagnosis in fibromyalgia in children and adolescents. Pediatrics. 1992;90:523-8.

15. **Hsu V, Patella SJ, Sigal LH.** "Chronic Lyme disease" as the incorrect diagnosis in patients with fibromyalgia. Arthritis Rheum. 1993;36:1493-500.

16. **Dinerman H, Steere AC.** Lyme disease associated with fibromyalgia. Ann Intern Med. 1992;117:281-5.

17. **Lightfoot RW Jr, Luft BJ, Rahn DW, et al.** Treatment of "possible Lyme disease": a practical policy position of the American College of Rheumatology and the Infectious Disease Society of America based on cost-benefit analysis. Ann Intern Med. 1993;119:503-9.

18. **Bennett RM.** Beyond fibromyalgia: ideas on etiology and treatment. J Rheumatol. 1989;16 (Suppl 19):185-91.

19. **Moldofsky H, Scarisbrick P.** Induction of neurasthenic musculoskeletal pain syndrome by selective sleep stage deprivation. Psychosom Med. 1976;38:35-44.

20. **Montgomery RR, Nathanson MH, Malawista SE.** The fate of *Borrelia burgdorferi*, the agent for Lyme disease, in mouse macrophages. J Immunol. 1993;150:909-15.

21. **Klempner MS, Noring R, Rogers RA.** Invasion of skin fibroblasts by the Lyme disease spirochete, *Borrelia burgdorferi*. J Infect Dis. 1993;167:1074-81.

22. **Haupl T, Hahn G, Rittig M, et al.** Persistence of *Borrelia burgdorferi* in ligamentous tissue from a patient with chronic Lyme borreliosis. Arthritis Rheum. 1993;36:1621-6.

23. **Stanek G, Klein J, Bittner R, et al.** Isolation of *Borrelia burgdorferi* from the myocardium of a patient with long-standing cardiomyopathy. N Engl J Med. 1990;322:249-53.

24. **Preac-Mursic V, Weber K, Pfister HW, et al.** Survival of *Borrelia burgdorferi* in antibiotically treated patients with Lyme borreliosis. Infection. 1989;17:355-9.

25. **Sigal LH.** The immunology and potential mechanisms of immunopathogenesis of Lyme disease. Annu Rev Immunol. 1997;15:63-92.

26. **Habicht GS, Beck G, Benach JL, et al.** Lyme disease spirochetes induce human and murine interleukin 1 production. J Immunol. 1985;134:3147-54.

27. **Habicht GS, Katona LI, Benach JL.** Cytokines and the pathogenesis of neuroborreliosis: *Borrelia burgdorferi* induces glioma cells to secrete interleukin-6. J Infect Dis. 1991;164:568-74.

28. **Yssel H, Shanafelt MC, Soderberg C, et al.** *Borrelia burgdorferi* activates T helper type 1–like T cell subsets in Lyme arthritis. J Exp Med. 1991;174:593-601.

29. **Gondolf KB, Mihatsch M, Curschellas E, et al.** Induction of experimental allergic arthritis with outer surface proteins of *Borrelia burgdorferi*. Arthritis Rheum. 1994;37:1070-7

30. **Meier C, Grahmann F, Engelhardt A, Dumas M.** Peripheral nerve disorders in Lyme-Borreliosis: nerve biopsy studies from eight cases. Acta Neuropathol. 1989;79:271-8.

31. **Duray PH.** Clinical pathologic correlations of Lyme disease. Rev Infect Dis. 1989;11:S1487-93.

32. **Sigal LH.** Lyme disease: Primum non nocere [editorial]. J Infect Dis. 1995;171:423-4.

33. **Weyand CM, Goronzy JJ.** Immune responses to *Borrelia burgdorferi* in patients with reactive arthritis. Arthritis Rheum. 1989;32:1057-64.

34. **Behar SM, Porcelli SA.** Mechanisms of autoimmune disease induction: the role of the immune response to microbial pathogens. Arthritis Rheum. 1995;38:458-76.

35. **Sigal LH.** Cross-reactivity between *Borrelia burgdorferi* flagellin and a human axonal 64,000 molecular weight protein. J Infect Dis. 1993;167:1372-8.

36. **Dai Z, Lackland H, Stein S, Li Q, et al.** Molecular mimicry in Lyme disease: monoclonal antibody H9724 to *Borrelia burgdorferi* flagellin specifically detects chaperonin-HSP60. Biochim Biophys Acta. 1993;1181:97-100.

37. **Sigal LH, Williams S.** A monoclonal antibody to *Borrelia burgdorferi's* flagellin modifies neuroblastoma cell neuritogenesis in vitro: a possible role for auto-immunity in the neuropathy of Lyme disease. Infect Immun. 1997; 65:1722-8.

38. **Sigal LH.** Pitfalls in the diagnosis and management of Lyme disease. Special Article. Arthritis Rheum. 1997 (In press).

39. **Spach DH, Liles WC, Campbell GL, et al.** Tick-borne diseases in the United States. N Engl J Med. 1993;329:936-47.

40. **Pruthi RK, Marshall WF, Wiltsie JC, Persing DH.** Human babesiosis. Mayo Clin Proc. 1995;70:853-62.

41. **Meldrum SC, Birkhead GS, White DJ, et al.** Human babesiosis in New York State: an epidemiological description of 136 cases. Clin Infect Dis. 1992;15:1019-23.

42. **Bakken JS, Dumler JS, Chen SM, et al.** Human granulocytic ehrlichiosis in the upper Midwest United States: a new species emerging? JAMA. 1994;272:212-8.

43. **Sigal LH.** The social and financial costs of the mismanagement of Lyme disease. Arch Intern Med. 1996; 156:1493-1500.

44. **Ettestad PJ, Campbell Gl, Welbel SF, et al.** Biliary complications in the treatment of unsubstantiated Lyme disease. J Infect Dis. 1995;171:356-61.

KEY REFERENCES

Hsu V, Patella SJ, Sigal LH. "Chronic Lyme disease" as the incorrect diagnosis in patients with fibromyalgia. Arthritis Rheum. 1993;36:1493-500.

Discusses how "chronic Lyme disease" may in fact be fibromyalgia, with the fibromyalgia being the real cause of the symptoms of musculoskeletal achiness, fatigue, and cognitive dysfunction reported by some patients.

Shadick NA, Phillips CB, Logigian EL, et al. The long-term clinical outcomes of Lyme disease: a population-based retrospective cohort study. Ann Intern Med. 1994;121:560-7.

Describes the long-term consequences of Lyme disease. Prior severe manifestations of Lyme disease do not predispose to the subsequent episode being remarkably worse—on the contrary, the previous exposure may actually ameliorate the second course of infection.

Sigal LH. Persisting complaints attributed to Lyme disease: Possible mechanisms and implications for management. Am J Med. 1994;96:365-74.

A proposed set of explanations for the persistence of symptoms after adequate antibiotic treatment for Lyme disease. Most such patients have no clinical evidence of ongoing infection and no objective evidence of Lyme disease.

Sigal LH. The social and financial costs of the mismanagement of Lyme disease. Arch Intern Med. 1997;156:1493-500.

Discusses the financial costs as well as the the emotional burden related to the diagnosis of "chronic Lyme disease."

Sigal LH. Pitfalls in the diagnosis and management of Lyme disease. Arthritis Rheum. 1997 (In press).

Discusses problems in approaches taken in diagnosis and management, highlighting incorrect use and interpretation of serologic testing.

Steere AC, Taylor E, McHugh GL, Logigian EL. The overdiagnosis of Lyme disease. JAMA. 1993;269:1812-6.

Describes the clinical experience at a regional referral center, showing that most patients seen at such centers did not have Lyme disease at the time of evaluation and that many probably never had Lyme disease, despite being diagnosed as having Lyme disease.

9

■ ■ ■

Lyme Disease Vaccine: Current Status

Robert T. Schoen, MD

Erol Fikrig, MD

The growing importance of Lyme disease in the United States has stimulated interest in the development of a safe and effective vaccine. First recognized in 1975, Lyme disease is now the most common vector-borne illness in the United States (1). Since 1982, when surveillance was initiated by the Centers for Disease Control and Prevention (CDC), there has been a nineteen-fold increase in reported cases. Most cases in North America occur in the coastal northeastern states (Massachusetts to Virginia), the Midwest (Minnesota and Wisconsin), and the western states (California, Oregon, and parts of Nevada). If a successful vaccine is developed, the distribution of the illness will strongly influence appropriate vaccine candidates.

Beyond North America, Lyme disease has been found in Europe, Russia, China, Japan, and Australia (2). As the widespread geographic distribution of Lyme disease has been recognized, antigenic diversity among different isolates of *Borrelia burgdorferi* from various geographic locations has also been appreciated. Significant heterogeneity among *B. burgdorferi* from the same geographic site, particularly in Europe, has been demonstrated (3).

Nucleic acid hybridization studies suggest that three new species of *B. burgdorferi* should be recognized—*B. burgdorferi* sensu stricto, *Borrelia afzelli,* and *Borrelia garinii* (4). *Borrelia burgdorferi* sensu stricto is dominant in North America, but all three species are seen in European sites. In considering potential vaccine candidates, the effectiveness of cross-protection between species and within different strains of the same species will need to be determined.

Current Preventive Measures

Currently available preventive measures to protect against Lyme disease are unsatisfactory (5). Residents of endemic areas may benefit from the use of repellents, protective clothing (light-colored clothing makes ticks easier to identify), and self-inspection for ticks, because ticks removed within 24 hours after attachment are relatively unlikely to transmit disease (6). These measures are cumbersome, however, and unlikely to be employed by most people.

Controversy exists as to whether asymptomatic persons should be given prophylactic antibiotic treatment after deer tick bites (7). Although infection rates among ixodid ticks from endemic areas are high (typically 10% to 35%), the likelihood of acquiring Lyme disease after a deer tick bite in an endemic area is much lower, presumably because in experimental studies in rodents, ticks often must remain attached for more than 48 hours for effective transmission of infection to occur. Prophylactic antibiotic treatment has a small risk of adverse effects, and in controlled clinical trials, such treatment has not proved to be of benefit (7).

For the community as a whole, currently available preventative measures attempt to reduce the prevalence of ixodid ticks by interruption of the tick life cycle. Habitat destruction, such as burning vegetation, spraying acaricides, distribution of acaricide-impregnated cotton balls to destroy ticks on reservoir mice, or reducing deer populations, has been attempted. These measures, however, are expensive, inefficient, and harmful to the environment (5). For these reasons, a safe and effective Lyme disease vaccine is desirable.

Experimental Vaccine Development

It is perhaps surprising that only 20 years after the clinical description of Lyme disease as a newly recognized illness (at least in North America; as the characteristic skin lesion, erythema migrans, was described in Europe in 1909) (8), vaccine development has already progressed to phase III human trials. Although the outcome of these and other clinical studies remains to be determined, progress in the laboratory during the past 10 years in several areas has allowed the development of candidate Lyme disease vaccines.

Immune Recognition of Spirochetal Antigens

Once the Lyme disease agent, *B. burgdorferi,* was identified, it became possible to culture the organisms in a complex liquid medium called Barbour-Stoenner-Kelly medium (2). It is relatively easy to obtain a primary isolate of *B. burgdorferi* from ticks. Unfortunately, it is more difficult to do so from patients.

In culture medium, *B. burgdorferi* expresses an abundant outer-surface protein A (OspA; molecular mass, 31 kd), a species-specific lipoprotein which, along with flagellin (molecular mass, 41 kd), accounts for approximately one third of total spirochete protein (9). More than 30 other proteins have also been identified (10), including OspB, OspC, P39, OspD, OspE, and OspF.

In early experimental models of infection in which animals were challenged with relatively large doses (10^7) of cultured spirochetes via syringe inoculation, antibodies developed within 2 weeks against the flagellin, P39, and OspC components, followed soon after by reactivity against OspA and OspB (11). In contrast, human patients with naturally acquired Lyme disease either do not seroconvert to OspA, seroconvert with low antibody titers, or seroconvert only several months after the onset of infection.

The lack of OspA immune recognition during naturally acquired infection is not unique to humans. Rhesus monkeys, dogs, mice, and hamsters with tick-borne infection do not seroconvert to OspA, even though they do so with syringe inoculation of spirochetes (12). It has been demonstrated that this difference in OspA immune recognition is dependent on the dose of *B. burgdorferi* administered, not the source of spirochetes. When syringe inoculation uses low doses (10^2 spirochetes), the host response resembles natural infection in which OspA immune recognition is weak (12).

Several factors may explain the limited host response to OspA during natural infection. Tick-borne infection transmits only a small number of spirochetes to the skin, perhaps less than 1,000. During feeding, ticks produce saliva which introduces antihomeostatic, anti-inflammatory, and immunosuppressant substances into the skin. As a result of these tick-mediated effects on the host, spirochetes may evade local destruction in skin, replicate, and disseminate via the bloodstream or lymphatics (5).

Recent experiments sampling *B. burgdorferi* from the midgut of unfed and fed ticks demonstrate that the recovered spirochetes produced OspA in the unfed state, but following a blood meal, *B. burgdorferi* that migrate from the tick midgut to salivary glands do not express OspA (13). Moreover, production of OspC, another outer-surface protein that stimulates an immune response early in human infection, is increased after the tick has become engorged (14). The switch to OspC is temperature-dependent, usually occurring at 32 °C to 37 °C degrees, but not at temperatures 24 °C or lower.

These two experimental stimuli—tick feeding and an increase in temperature—may trigger a major alteration of the spirochetal outer membrane, which allows survival in a warm-blooded host. Therefore an OspA-vaccine is arthropod-specific, because it exerts its action solely in the midgut of an unengorged tick (13).

Animal Model

In 1986, active immunization of hamsters with a single dose of an inactivated B. burgdorferi whole-cell lysate vaccine conveyed protection against high doses of a homologous strain (15). Protection was greater when challenge occurred 30 days after vaccination compared to 90 days after vaccination. Early studies in the mouse failed to establish infection or demonstrate reproducible pathologic change, but in 1990, C3H/HeJ mice were reported to develop both significant arthritis and cardiac lesions (16). Spirochetes could be cultured from blood and joint fluid, and arthritis and carditis, which appeared at to 2 to 3 weeks, persisted for up to 1 year. These mice did not develop neurologic disease or a characteristic skin rash. Both the arthritis and carditis were found to be genotype-dependent, because other strains of mice developed less severe infection, and age-dependent, because younger mice had more severe disease.

Animal Vaccine Experiments

After the molecular identification of OspA as a major surface antigen, the demonstration that an inactivated whole-cell B. burgdorferi vaccine was protective in hamsters, and the development of a mouse model of Lyme disease in the C3H/HeJ mouse, a monotypic recombinant OspA (rOspA) vaccine was shown to be protective in the C3H/HeJ mouse model (17). Using the polymerase chain reaction and primers designed from full-length OspA and OspB sequences from strain B31, the capacity of recombinant fusion proteins to induce protection in the C3H/HeJ mouse was demonstrated (17).

Active immunization with rOspA or rOspB glutathione transferase fusion proteins in complete Freund adjuvant resulted in the production of high antibody titers (1:1000—or greater by immunoblot) to these surface antigens. OspA-vaccinated mice that were challenged by syringe inoculation with 10^4 B. burgdorferi organisms 5 weeks after vaccination had 100% protection against infection and disease as measured by culture and histopathologic examination. OspB vaccination was also fully protective at lower inoculation doses of 10^4 organisms. Passive immunization with rOspA antibodies was also shown to be protective, indicating that the humoral response is sufficient for immunity. The contribution of the cellular immune response to protection has yet to be clearly established (17).

In these experiments, animals were killed 14 days after challenge inoculation. In human Lyme disease, spirochetes have been visualized or cultured from blood, synovial fluid, and cerebrospinal fluid samples, cardiac tissue specimens, and dermatologic lesions for a long time after initial infection. In one case report, spirochetes were isolated from a patient with acrodermatitis chronica atrophicans 10 years after initial infection (18). In the C3H/HeJ mouse model, spirochetes may be isolated from cultures of blood, spleen, and bladder for up to 1 year after infection, even in the presence of antibody to *B. burgdorferi*. In experiments in which vaccinated mice were killed 60, 120, and 180 days after challenge, the protective effect of rOspA vaccination was demonstrated both against infection (measured by culture) and disease (assessed by histopathologic examination) (19). OspA-vaccinated mice that were challenged with spirochetes 60 to 150 days after vaccination were also protected from infection and disease (19).

The protective effect of OspA vaccination in these experiments has been confirmed using various preparations of OspA or monoclonal antibodies directed against this antigen. One system uses bacille Calmette-Guérin (BCG) as a shuttle vector, allowing oral vaccination (20). It has also been demonstrated that the protective epitopes on OspA are mainly found in the carboxy terminal third of OspA, because monoclonal antibodies against OspA that protect mice against infection bind peptides within this region (21).

Mechanisms of Protection

Protection for both OspA- and OspB-based vaccines has been found to be spirochete dose–dependent in syringe challenge experiments, but protection occurring after OspA immunization against tick-transmitted infection has been shown to be almost completely effective in the mouse model. This is because tick-borne infection introduces the more complex biology of natural vector transmission, which includes several factors: the inoculant size, the possibility that anti-inflammatory properties of tick saliva may enhance transmission, and the likelihood that vector-borne *B. burgdorferi* differs from organisms propagated *in vitro*.

In addition, the 2-year life cycle of ixodid ticks is complex and therefore potentially vulnerable to manipulation; their life cycle could thus be exploited to reduce the risk of human infection (5). *Borrelia burgdorferi* remains dormant in the tick midgut for much of the life cycle and becomes activated only after attachment of the tick to a host. Spirochetes then multiply within the midgut of the tick and move to the salivary gland, where they enter the mammalian host via salivary fluid (22). At each stage in the life cycle—larval, nymphal, and adult—a single feeding is necessary to proceed to the next stage. In the eastern United States, the preferred host for both the larval and nymphal stage of *Ixodes scapularis* is the white-footed mouse, *Peromyscus leucopus*. White-tailed deer are the preferred host for the adult stage (2).

The reactivation of spirochetes in the midgut after tick feeding probably takes 48 hours and explains why Lyme disease is unlikely to be transmitted until after engorgement. It may also explain the somewhat unexpected finding that active immunization with rOspA protects mice against-tick-borne spirochetal infection by destroying *B. burgdorferi* within the midgut of ticks feeding on vaccinated mice even before the spirochete enters the mammalian host (23). Immunofluorescent studies demonstrate elimination of viable spirochetes in the midgut of the ticks feeding on OspA-vaccinated mice, but spirochetes in ticks feeding on control mice are not affected. Spirochetes remain in the midgut long enough during tick feeding to allow antibody to enter the gut and kill the organism before reactivation.

This finding suggests that an OspA vaccine has a unique dual mode of action (13). Spirochetes are killed within the tick midgut before transmission to the vaccinated host. In the event that this mechanism is bypassed (for example, in syringe inoculation experiments), OspA antibodies in the host kill the organism directly (23).

Passive immunization experiments with hyperimmune serum also suggest that protection occurs primarily because of spirochete destruction within the tick and not within the mammalian host (24). Mice are protected when infused with hyperimmune serum no later than 1 day after infected ticks are allowed to attach. At this time, spirochetes in the midgut begin to express OspA. If hyperimmune serum is infused 3 to 5 days after tick attachment, up to 100% of mice became infected because spirochetes in the salivary glands are no longer expressing OspA. This suggests that spirochetal antibody is protective only if administered before spirochetes enter the skin of the host (24).

Other outer-surface proteins have been studied for their protective effect. OspC was found to be protective in gerbils and mice (25). Although OspC appears to be an important antigen early in human infection, possibly facilitating the transition of the spirochete to the higher temperature of the mammalian host, OspC is a highly heterogeneous protein, potentially limiting its usefulness as a vaccine candidate (5). OspF is very weakly protective, and the immune response to OspE is not protective (26).

One of the most important questions concerning the feasibility of a human Lyme disease vaccine is whether an OspA-based vaccine developed with one strain of *B. burgdorferi* will be widely cross-protective. The division of *B. burgdorferi* into three distinctive genospecies and the demonstration of antigenic differences in OspA and OspB in these different groups add to this concern. Isolates of the Lyme disease spirochete frequently differ antigenetically, even when taken from the same geographic site. Variability mainly affects the outer-surface proteins and is greatest in European isolates. In addition, mutations, frame shifts, and homologous recombination between OspA and OspB have been demonstrated, and spirochetes that lack the 49-kd linear plasmid that encodes OspA and B have been identified (5).

Initial studies evaluating cross-protection were discouraging. For example, in syringe challenge studies, vaccination with OspA-N40 did not protect mice against heterologous spirochetes (strain 25015) in which OspA differs by 40 amino acids (27). These studies suggested that protective immunity may be strain- or site-specific and that a monotypic recombinant antigen may be of limited value as a vaccine.

Experiments evaluating whether OspA or OspB immunization protects mice from *B. burgdorferi* infection transmitted by tick-borne infection have been more encouraging. Ticks collected from different taxonomic groups in the United States and Europe show a greater degree of cross-protection in tick challenge experiments than would have been predicted in syringe challenge experiments (3). These studies suggest that cross-protection must be assessed by tick challenge, not syringe challenge, but the final answer to this question must await human clinical trials.

Clinical Vaccine Trials

Animal Vaccine

In 1990 a whole-cell, chemically inactivated *B. burgdorferi* vaccine with a proprietary adjuvant (*Borrelia burgdorferi* bacterin; Lymevax, Fort Dodge Laboratories, Fort Dodge, Iowa) was provisionally licensed by the U.S. Department of Agriculture for use in dogs (28). This animal vaccine was fully licensed in 1992, but little information about its safety and effectiveness is available.

The use of a whole-cell vaccine in humans is also limited by concern that there might be possible autoimmunity to numerous cross-reactive bacterial epitopes (5). In one study, hamsters vaccinated with a whole-cell preparation of formalin-inactivated *B. burgdorferi* developed severe destructive arthritis when challenged with homologous *B. burgdorferi* (29). It should be noted that serious adverse reactions in dogs to the commercially available whole-cell vaccine have not been reported. An additional concern has been the use of the Fort Dodge animal vaccine by humans either to prevent infection or treat "chronic Lyme disease" (30). The long-term safety of use of this vaccine in this manner is unknown.

Human Vaccine

Several studies to assess the safety and efficacy of Lyme disease vaccines intended for human use and based on rOspA have been completed. In a phase II study, 350 healthy adults with no history of infection, residing on three New England islands on which Lyme disease is highly endemic, were enrolled in a randomized, double-blind, placebo-controlled, dose-ranging trial. Three doses (3, 10, and 30 µg) of the rOspA vaccine were given. No serious adverse events related to the vaccine occurred. General reactions such as fever, fatigue, and headache occurred with fewer than 30% of injections. Solicited local reactions were frequent but mild. Anti-OspA antibodies were detected by enzyme-linked immunosorbent assay (ELISA) in more than 97% of study participants who received the vaccine, and immunogenicity correlated with the vaccine dose. When suspected Lyme disease cases were unblinded, vaccine efficacy against laboratory-confirmed clinical Lyme disease was 100%. By less strict criteria, there was 56% to 78% efficacy against "symptomatic Lyme disease" or serologic detection (31).

In a second study, the safety and immunogenicity of three injections of three doses of the vaccine (3, 10, and 30 µg) were evaluated in patients with previous clinical and laboratory evidence of Lyme disease. Again, all three dosages of vaccine were well tolerated. Arthralgia occurred after three infections but was minor and self limited. All patients developed an increase in IgG ELISA titers to whole-cell B. burgdorferi and OspA, which was vaccine dose dependent. This study suggests that it is safe to vaccinate persons who have a history of previous Lyme disease (32). Based on this study and other safety data as well as the preliminary evidence of efficacy in the New England island trial, a larger phase III has been conducted to evaluate the effectiveness of this Lyme disease vaccine.

Two double-blinded phase III trials have also been completed, and efficacy and safety data have been presented in abstract form. Both studies identified participants residing in areas where Lyme disease is endemic (incidence, 0.5% to 3%). In one study, SmithKline Beecham Pharmaceuticals has evaluated the safety and effectiveness of an rOspA vaccine based on the German ZS7 B. burgdorferi senso structo strain (33). This rOspA is expressed in Escherichia coli as a lipoprotein and is highly purified to remove nonrecombinant contaminants. The adjuvant is aluminum hydroxide (SmithKline Beecham Pharmaceuticals, Inc., data on file). The SmithKline Beecham trial was a multicenter double-blind placebo controlled trial of 10,936 participants aged 15 to 70 years. Participants received three injections of adjuvanated L-OspA vaccine or placebo on a 0-, 1-, and 12-month schedule. Suspected Lyme disease was demonstrated by culture, polymerase chain reaction, and/or serologic testing. Asymptomatic infection was also assessed by serologic testing at 12 and 20 months after study entry in all participants. Vaccine efficacy was 50% after two doses and 79% after three doses. Vaccine efficacy was also high for asymptomatic infection (83% after two doses, 100% after three doses). Local and general adverse events were slightly higher in the vaccine group, but these were mild to moderate and tended to be self-limited.

Another phase III trial has evaluated an OspA lipoprotein vaccine that has been developed by Connaught Laboratories (34). This is also an rOspA vaccine expressed by *E. coli*. A safety and immunogenicity study of this vaccine in 36 healthy adult volunteers was published prior to the phase III trial (35). In this earlier study, volunteers were randomly assigned to receive two 10-μg doses of the OspA vaccine, vaccine absorbed to aluminum hydroxide, or a placebo. Study participants in the OspA vaccine group received a third dose. The most common reactions, local pain and tenderness at the injection site, were mild and did not increase after the second and third dose. Two doses of both vaccine formulations elicited high titer antibodies and inhibited replication of *B. burgdorferi* in vitro. The phase III trial was based on this and other data.

In the Connaught trial, vaccine efficacy and safety were also demonstrated. Participants received vaccines on a 0-, 1-, and 12-month schedule. Lyme disease was diagnosed clinically and serologically. Vaccine efficacy in adults younger than 59 years old after two or three doses was 82% and 100%, respectively. Efficacy was somewhat lower in persons older than 60 years (75% after the third dose). The frequency of adverse events (including neurologic and rheumatic adverse events or serious adverse events) in the vaccine group did not significantly exceed that of the placebo group.

Each of these vaccines will be submitted to United States Food and Drug Administration for approval so that an rOspA-based Lyme disease vaccine may be available for clinical use in the near future.

Conclusion

Only 20 years after the recognition of Lyme disease as a distinct clinical entity in the United States, the causative organism, *B. burgdorferi*, has been identified. An experimental animal model has allowed Lyme disease vaccine research to proceed such that two rOspA lipoprotein vaccines are in phase III clinical trials. Preliminary results from these studies demonstrate vaccine efficacy and safety, and a new public health approach to the containment of Lyme disease may be possible.

■   ■   ■

Key Points

- In a mouse model, vaccination with *Borrelia burgdorferi* rOspA protects against experimental Lyme disease.

- The mechanism of protection may be antibody-mediated killing of spirochetes in the tick midgut before their transmission to the vaccinated host.

Because of promising experimental results, two rOspA Lyme disease vaccines for humans have completed stage III clinical trials.

▪   ▪   ▪

REFERENCES

1. **CDC.** Emerging infectious disease. Lyme disease: United States, 1992–1993. MMWR. 1994;43:564-72.

2. **Steere AC.** Lyme disease. N Engl J Med. 1989;321:586-96.

3. **Fikrig E, Telford SR, Wallich R, et al.** Vaccination against Lyme disease caused by diverse *Borrelia burgdorferi.* J Exp Med. 1995;181: 215-21.

4. **Baranton G, Postic D, Saint Girons I, et al.** Delineation of *Borrelia burgdorferi* sensu stricto, *Borrelia garinii* sp. nov., and group VS461 associated with Lyme borreliosis. Int J Syst Bacteriol. 1992:42:378-83.

5. **Telford SR, Fikrig E.** Progress towards a vaccine for Lyme disease. Clin Immunother. 1995;4:49-60.

6. **Piesman J, Mather TN, Sinsky RJ, Spielman A.** Duration of tick attachment and *Borrelia burgdorferi* transmission. J Clin Microbiol. 1987;25:557-8.

7. **Shapiro ED, Gerber MA, Holabird NB, et al.** A controlled trial of antimicrobial prophylaxis for Lyme disease after deer tick bites. N Engl J Med. 1992;327: 1769-73.

8. Erythema chronicum migrans. Acta Derm Venereol (Stockh) 1921;2:120-5.

9. **Coleman JL, Benach JL.** Isolation of antigenic components from the Lyme disease spirochete: their role in early diagnosis. J Infect Dis. 1987;155:756-65.

10. **Craft JE, Fischer DK, Shimamoto GT, Steere AC.** Antigens of *Borrelia burgdorferi* recognized during Lyme disease: appearance of a new immunogloblin M response and expansion of the immunoglobin G response late in the illness. J Clin Invest. 1986;78:934-9.

11. **Barthold SW, Persing DH, Armstrong AL, Peeples RA.** Kinetics of *Borrelia burgdorferi* dissemination and evolution of disease after intradermal inoculation of mice. Am J Pathol. 1991;139:263-73.

12. **Barthold SW, Fikrig E, Bockenstedt LK, Persing DH.** Circumvention of outer surface protein A immunity by host-adapted *Borrelia burgdorferi.* Infect Immun. 1995;63:2255-61.

13. **de Silva AM, Telford SR III, Brunet LR, et al.** *Borrelia burgdorferi* OspA is an arthropod-specific transmission blocking Lyme disease vaccine. J Exp Med. 1996;183:271-5.

14. **Schwan TG, Piesman J, Golde WT, et al.** Induction of an outer surface protein on *Borrelia burgdorferi* during feeding. Proc Natl Acad Sci U S A. 1995;92:2909-13.

15. **Johnson RC, Kodner C, Russell M.** Active immunization of hamsters against experimental infection with *Borrelia burgdorferi* . Infect Immun. 1986;54:897-8.

16. **Barthold SW, Beck DS, Hansen GM, et al.** Lyme borrelosis in selected strains and ages of laboratory mice. J Infect Dis. 1990;162:133-8.

17. **Fikrig E, Barthold SW, Kantor FS, Flavell RA.** Protection of mice against the Lyme disease agent by immunizing with recombinant OspA. Science. 1990;250: 553-6.

18. **Asbrink E, Hovmark A.** Successful cultivation of spirochetes from skin lesions of patients with erythema chronicum migrans Afzelius and acrodermatitis chronica atrophicans. Acta Pathol Microbiol Scand. 1985;93:161-3.

19. **Fikrig E, Barthold SW, Kantor FS, Flavell RA.** Long-term protection of mice from Lyme disease by vaccination with OspA. Infect Immun. 1992;60:773-7.

20. **Hanson MS, Lapcevich CV, Haun SL.** Progress on the development of the live BCG recombinant vaccine vehicle for combined vaccine delivery. Ann N Y Acad Sci. 1995;754:214-21.

21. **Sears JE, Fikrig E, Nakagawa TY, et al.** Molecular mapping of OspA-mediated immunity against *Borrelia burgdorferi,* the agent of Lyme disease. J Immunol. 1991;147:1995-2000.

22. **Zung JL, Lewewgrub S, Rudzinska MA.** Time structured evidence for the penetration of the Lyme spirochete *Borrelia burgdorferi* through the gut tissues and salivary glands in *Ioxides dammini.* Can J Zool. 1989;67:1737-48.

23. **Fikrig E, Telford SR III, Barthold SW, et al.** Elimination of *Borrelia burgdorferi* from vector ticks feeding on OspA-immunized mice. Proc Natl Acad Sci U S A. 1992;89;5418-21.

24. **Shih CM, Spielman A, Telford SR.** Short report: mode of action of protective immunity to Lyme disease spirochetes. Am J Trop Med Hyg. 1995;52:72-4.

25. **Preac-Mursic V, Wilske B, Patsouris E, et al.** Active immunization with pC protein of *Borrelia burgdorferi* protects gerbils against *B. burgdorferi* infection. Infection. 1992;20:342-9.

26. **Nguyen TP, Lam TT, Barthold SW, et al.** Partial destruction of *Borrelia burgdorferi* within ticks that engorged on OspE- or OspF-immunized mice. Infect Immun. 1994;62;2079-84.

27. **Fikrig E, Barthold SW, Persing DH, et al.** *Borrelia burgdorferi* strain 25015: characterization of outer surface protein A and vaccination against infection. J Immunol. 1992;148;2256-60.

28. **Chu HJ, Chavez LG Jr, Blumer BM, et al.** Immunogenuity and efficacy study of a commercial *Borrelia burgdorferi* bacterin. J Am Vet Med Assoc. 1992;201:403-11.

29. **Lim LC, England DM, DuChateau, et al.** Development of destructive arthritis in vaccinated hamsters challenged with *Borrelia burgdorferi.* Infect Immun. 1994;62:2825-33.

30. **Feaga WP.** Self dosing of the Borrelia vaccine by veterinarians [abstract]. Presented at Lyme Disease: State of the Art. Seventh Annual Scientific Conference of Lyme Borreliosis and Other Spirochetal and Tick-Borne Diseases. April 1994. Stamford, Connecticut. The Lyme Borreliosis Foundation. 1994.

31. **Telford SR, Krause P, Meurice F, et al.** Safety and immunogenicity of a candidate of Lyme disease vaccine in residents of endemic New England sites. Presented at the 35th Interscience Conference of Antimicrobial Agents and Chemotherapy (ICAAC), San Francisco, 1995. G31:164.

32. **Schoen RT, Meurice F, Brunet CM, et al.** Safety and immunogenicity of an outer surface protein A vaccine in subjects with previous Lyme disease. J Infect Dis. 1995;172;1321-9.

33. **Steere AC, Sikand VK, Schoen RT, et al.** Successful vaccination for Lyme disease (LD) using a recombinant, adjuvanted *Borrelia burgdorferi* outer surface lipoprotein A (L-OspA) vaccine. In: Programs and Abstracts of the 35th Annual Meeting of the Infectious Disease Society of America, 1997.

34. **Sigal LH, Adler Klein D, et al.** Multicenter efficacy trial of a prophylactic recombinant *Borrelia burgdorferi* outer surface protein A vaccine for Lyme disease; 422. In: Programs and Abstracts of the 35th Annual Meeting of the Infectious Disease Society of America, 1997.

35. **Keller D, Koster FT, Marsk DH, et al.** Safety and immunogenicity of a recombinant outer surface protein A Lyme vaccine. JAMA. 1994;271:1764-8.

KEY REFERENCES

CDC. Emerging infectious disease. Lyme disease—United States, 1992–1993. MMWR. 1994;43:564–72.

An rOspA vaccine protects against Lyme disease in the mouse model.

Kellet D, Koster FT, Marks DH, *et al*. Safety and immunogenicity of an rOspA Lyme vaccine. JAMA. 1994;271:1764–8.

The first published phase II clinical trial data about Lyme disease vaccine safety and immunogenicity.

Schoen RT, Meurice F, Brunet CM. Safety and immunogenicity of an outer surface protein A vaccine in subjects with previous Lyme disease. J Infect Dis. 1995;172;1321–9.

Vaccination of study participants with a previous history of Lyme disease was found to be safe in this phase II clinical trial.

Telford SR, Fikrig E. Progress towards a vaccine for Lyme disease. Clin Immunother. 1995;4:49–60.

A review summarizing the experimental studies that led to vaccine development.

10

■ ■ ■

Use of the Laboratory in the Confirmation and Management of Lyme Disease

Leonard H. Sigal, MD

The clinical features of Lyme disease are well described (1). No longer is infection with *Borrelia burgdorferi* known as "the great imitator" (2); we now know that most cases fall within well-defined clinical syndromes (3). Thus, the diagnosis of Lyme disease can usually be made on the basis of objective clinical findings alone, with serologic testing used solely to confirm the diagnosis.

In many infectious diseases, such as pneumonia or urinary tract infections, it is usually possible to isolate the pathogen. Unfortunately, in Lyme disease, this approach is not practical, owing to the paucity of organisms present in affected tissues and the fastidious culture requirements of the organism. Attempting to identify the organism by histopathologic or immunologic techniques also is not very helpful. We depend on measurement of the immune response to the organism for indirect evidence of exposure. This chapter describes the most common serologic techniques currently used and summarizes the investigational techniques whose value has not yet been proved.

The Human Humoral Immune Response

Ten to fourteen days after exposure to a new foreign protein, the human body produces IgM antibodies. Shortly thereafter, IgG antibodies (and often IgA) are made, with the IgM levels either persisting or diminishing to baseline. This sequence is called the primary immune response, because it occurs after the initial, or primary, exposure to the protein.

On subsequent exposure to the same protein, a secondary response (also called memory or anamnestic response) occurs, which is different from the primary immune response. The IgG response occurs more rapidly, and the IgM response is briefer (4).

In all the antibody assays described, detection systems can identify IgM, IgA, and IgG antibodies, separately or in sum, by using different types of anti-human immunoglobulin reagents made in sheep or goats.

Current Testing to Confirm the Clinical Diagnosis of Lyme Disease

Indirect Immunofluorescence Assay

In the indirect immunofluorescence assay (IFA), the organism is fixed to a glass slide and the slide is flooded with a dilution of the serum to be tested. The unbound or excess serum is washed away. The slide is then flooded with a fluoresceinated anti-human antibody (i.e., an antibody against human immunoglobulin, usually made in a goat or sheep), which binds to the antibody–organism complexes. Once the excess antibody is washed away, the slide is dried and exposed to the wavelength of light which makes fluorescein glow, or fluoresce. *Borrelia burgdorferi* bound by antibody in the serum being tested will appear green.

The laboratory tests many normal sera to determine the highest dilution of normal serum that still gives a negative result; the test is set up so that in many laboratories, a 1:128 dilution is the upper limit of normal. Thus, the sample to be tested is diluted to 1:128 and tested; if the result is positive, sequential twofold dilutions are done until the test result is negative. The result is then reported as the highest dilution at which the assay remained positive.

The indirect immunofluoresence assay has limitations: It is difficult to do large numbers of IFAs at a time, and interpretation is very dependent on the technician's experience. IFA has been replaced in most laboratories by enzyme-linked immunosorbent assay (ELISA).

Enzyme-Linked Immunosorbent Assay

Enzyme-linked immunosorbent assay is currently the most common initial test to serologically confirm Lyme disease. ELISA is done using plastic "microtiter plates," which contain 96 small wells. The inside of each well is coated with a derivative of *B. burgdorferi* (e.g., a sonicated preparation or whole organism). Before test serum is added, the plate is "blocked" so that the plastic surface of the wells does not nonspecifically bind serum antibodies.

A set dilution of the serum to be tested is then added to a defined number of the wells and allowed to bind to the organism's antigens on the inner surface of the wells. An anti-human immunoglobulin which is conjugated to an enzyme is then added to the wells, which in turn binds the antibody–antigen complexes. After the unbound immunoglobulin has been washed away, a special substrate (known as a chromogen) for that enzyme is added and changes color when it is modified by the enzyme. The color generated is measured by an automatic ELISA plate-reader, and the amount of color is expressed as the "optical density" (OD).

ELISA results for that serum sample can then be reported with an upper limit of normal (statistically derived from results obtained by testing a large series of normal sera and usually equal to the mean plus 3 SD) as the ratio of the patient's OD to the "upper limit of normal;" or as the dilution of the patient serum that still exceeds an upper normal range.

Several samples can be tested by ELISA with ease and reproducibility. Nonetheless, because of the variation of *B. burgdorferi* in culture and the variability of techniques, results from ELISAs in different laboratories may vary.

Causes of False-Positive Results

False-positive results in ELISA are common. Cross-reacting antibodies can occur in patients with other spirochetal diseases, including other *Borrelia* infections (e.g., relapsing fever or even the cause of mild gingivitis), leptospirosis, or treponemal infections (e.g., syphilis), as well as with enteroviral or other viral illnesses and autoimmune diseases (e.g., systemic lupus erythematosus or rheumatoid arthritis) (5).

Many bacteria contain certain proteins that are closely related to homologous proteins in other organisms—for example, heat shock proteins or flagellin. A strong immune response to the heat shock protein or flagellin of a constituent of the gut flora or to a previous cause of urinary tract infection or pneumonia can bind to the *B. burgdorferi* within the well of the ELISA plate to cause a positive ELISA reading, even though there has been no exposure to *B. burgdorferi* and there is no diagnosis of current Lyme disease.

In addition, antibodies that bind to *B. burgdorferi* may be produced because of nonspecific activation of immunoglobulin production, known as polyclonal B-cell activation, found in association with infections with Epstein-Barr virus and certain parasites, notably malaria. In these examples, such activation can result in ELISA positivity unrelated to Lyme disease (6,7). The same phenomenon can be seen in chronic inflammatory diseases, such as nonspirochetal subacute bacterial endocarditis (8).

Also, the standard statistics used to define a "normal range" for ELISA results ensures that a certain percentage of normal people fall outside the normal range. By definition, in a normal population, if one defines the mean and takes a group within 2 SD of that mean, there will be a group "outside" the "normal range" defined by that 2 SD width. It is estimated that up to 5% of the normal population "test positive" for Lyme disease by ELISA (6,7), and a higher proportion may have positive test results in endemic areas, perhaps representing previous exposure.

The high frequency of false-positive test results is an excellent argument against screening serologic tests. With long-term experience with Western blot analysis, which can determine the presence of antibodies to specific constituents of B. burgdorferi, it became apparent that criteria could be developed by which positive ELISA results could be corroborated or refuted.

Western Blot

Also known as immunoblot, the Western blot procedure allows detection of antibodies to individual components of the organism and is therefore much more specific than ELISA. Western blot depends on a technique known as electrophoresis. A mixture of proteins (e.g., derived from B. burgdorferi) is placed in a trench at the top of a gel which contains many microscopic pores. The gel containing the trench is then placed in an electric field, and the proteins migrate through the pores. Each protein moves a distance dependent on its molecular mass. The end result of electrophoresis is that the borrelial proteins can be separated by molecular mass (designated in units called kilodaltons).

After electrophoresis is completed, the gel with the proteins separated is placed on the surface of a membrane, and the proteins are transferred to the membrane surface by means of an electric field. The conditions of the assay can be manipulated so that binding of serum antibodies to the proteins on the membrane surface occurs only with the specific protein against which the antibody was made. Detection of the antibody can be by ELISA or by use of a radioactive-tagged anti-human immunoglobulin, in which case the bound antibodies are detected on radiograph film.

The advantage of Western blot is that it detects binding of antibody only to its specific antigen. Low-level nonspecific binding, as is especially common with the IgM antibodies made in the primary immune response, is eliminated by the conditions of the assay. Studies correlating clinically diagnosed Lyme disease with patterns of reactivity in immunoblot have allowed criteria to be proposed by the Centers for Disease Control and Prevention [9,10] (Table 10.1). The current recommendation is that *all equivocal or positive ELISA results be corroborated by Western blot analysis*, in order to differentiate between false-positive and true-positive ELISA results.

Table 10.1   Criteria for Positive Western Blot Analysis in the Serologic Confirmation of Infection with *Borrelia burgdorferi* (Lyme disease)*

Disease Stage	Isotype Tested	Bands to be Considered
First few weeks of infection	IgM	Two of the eight following: 18-, 21-, 28-, 37-, 41-, 45-, 58-, 93-kd
		or
		Two of the three following: OspC (23), 39, 41[†]
After first few weeks of infection	IgG	Five of the ten following: 18-, 21-, 28-, 30-, 39-, 41-, 45-, 58-, 66-, 93-kd

Osp = outer-surface protein.
*Data from Dressler F, Whalen JA, Reinhardt BN, Steere AC. Western blotting in the serodiagnosis of Lyme disease. J Infect Dis. 1993;167:392-400.
[†]Alternate criteria for IgM reactivity, proposed by the Centers for Disease Control and Prevention [10] and now more widely adopted. Other points noted at that conference of the CDC were the need for standardization of antigen preparation and techniques.

Molecular biologic research into the structures of *B. burgdorferi* has identified multiple components of the organism (Table 10.2). More components of the organism are being identified, but the functions of these proteins and lipoproteins are not yet defined (11).

Cautions in the Interpretation of Serologic Tests

Several issues must be considered when interpreting serologic test results: 1) false-positive results, 2) false-negative results, 3) interlaboratory variation, and 4) the persistence of seropositivity.

False-Positive Results

In the absence of Western blot corroboration, an isolated positive ELISA should not be taken as serologic confirmation of the clinical diagnosis of Lyme disease. Bayes theorem can be used to appreciate the proper role of "diagnostic" tests. The theorem states that if the pre-test likelihood of a disease is high, the predictive value of a positive test result for that disease (i.e., a positive test result confirming that the disease is really present) is high. If, on the other hand, the pre-test likelihood of the disease is low (i.e., if the patient tested is from a nonendemic area or if it is more likely that the condition is a clinical syndrome dissimilar from Lyme disease), the positive predictive value is low: a positive test result is more likely to be a false-positive result than one truly indicative of Lyme disease.

Table 10.2   Some Identified Components of *Borrelia burgdorferi*

Name	Molecular Mass (kd)	Function or Homology
OspA*	31	
OspB	34	
OspC	21–24†	
BmpA (p39)	39	Serologic reactivity may be highly specific for Lyme disease
Flagellin	41	Motility component; strong homology with flagellins of other organisms
Heat shock	58, 60, 66, 72	Response to stress experienced by all living cells proteins; strong homology with heat shock proteins of other organisms

Osp = outer-surface protein.
*OspA, OspB, and OspC have been well characterized, and OspA and OspC may be useful in seroconfirmation of the diagnosis. Other Osps also have been identified: D, E, F, G, and H.
†The precise mass of OspC is dependent on the strain of *B. burgdorferi* being tested.

Thus, if one tests several patients with bilateral facial nerve palsy from an area endemic for Lyme disease, most of the positive ELISA tests are likely to represent immunologic confirmation of exposure to *B. burgdorferi*. However, if one were to screen people with isolated fatigue (an unlikely clinical scenario in Lyme disease), or all women at the start of their pregnancy, or all citizens of Havre, Montana (a nonendemic area), the odds are that a positive test result will be a false-positive and not indicative of Lyme disease.

Screening Serologic Tests
Some clinicians use serologic testing as a screening tool in clinical circumstances not suggestive of Lyme disease. The high frequency of both "atypical features of Lyme disease" and the failure of patients diagnosed in this manner to respond to antibiotic therapy in these practices suggest that diagnosis purely by serologic screening is poor practice. The financial consequences of treating all such persons who have false-positive test results for Lyme disease has been discussed (12). *It is crucial that the diagnosis of Lyme disease be based on the presence of objective findings, not merely on the basis of isolated subjective symptoms, even if associated with serologic reactivity.*

As noted, because serologic testing is often misused as a screening tool, there may be asymptomatic patients with serum antibodies to *B. burgdorferi* who present for evaluation. For the purposes of this discussion, let us assume that the patient in question has a positive ELISA confirmed by Western blot (if they have a positive ELISA but negative Western blot, they are not truly seropositive).

The first question is, What is the significance of such a result? Although some ascribe no importance to isolated seroreactivity, others, including our group, consider that these persons may have latent infection, analogous with latent syphilis. We prescribe 1 month of oral antibiotic therapy for these patients, the same regimen used for patients with other features of Lyme disease; the goal is to use a relatively benign therapy to prevent progression to later features of Lyme disease. This approach has never been subjected to scientific study and is merely a recommendation based on our experience (see Case 10.1).

False-Negative Results

Lack of Sensitivity in Early Lyme Disease
Exposure of a naive person (that is, someone not previously exposed) to a new protein antigen usually results in the production of measurable IgM within 10 to 14 days, followed by the production of measurable IgG antibodies within 2 weeks (4). In Lyme disease, however, antibodies may not

---

CASE 10.1   *A patient with nonspecific symptoms and "equivocal" serologic results who does not respond to antibiotic therapy*

A 28-year-old man presents with symptoms including headache, fatigue, confusion, numbness in his hands and feet, low back pain, neck pain, abdominal pain, nausea, occasional diarrhea, and difficulty in taking a deep breath. Fifteen months ago he was diagnosed by a local physician as having Lyme disease. Since then, he has been receiving intravenous or oral antibiotics or both with no more than a 1-week interval between treatments. He describes no improvement with this treatment.

Review of his medical records from the treating physician reveals that the results of the physical examination were normal at the outset and that the serologic response was positive: three samples from the first visit were sent to different laboratories and one was reported as equivocal (OD, 0.83 [normal <0.8, equivocal 0.8 to 1.2, and positive >1.2]). No immunoblot was done to confirm this ELISA result. The results of the current physical examination are also normal.

The patient is incredulous to hear that he probably never had Lyme disease. He leaves the office saying that he will simply have to find another doctor, one who is more "in tune" with Lyme disease than you, the disabusing clinician.

be detectable by ELISA for up to 6 to 8 weeks (and somewhat sooner by Western blot).

IgM typically appears 2 to 4 weeks after the onset of erythema migrans, peaks at 6 to 8 weeks, and declines to low levels after 4 to 6 months. IgG appears after 6 to 8 weeks, peaks at 4 to 6 months, and often remains elevated indefinitely despite therapy and resolution of symptoms.

The reason for the common delay in the appearance of measurable antibodies in Lyme disease is not known. It may be that the assays currently available are not sufficiently sensitive or that the antibodies are bound in immune complexes during the early stages of the disease (11).

The net effect is that as many as 50% of patients with early Lyme disease are "antibody-negative"—in a sense, producing a "false-negative" result. *Thus, serologic testing is not necessary or useful for diagnosis in the patient with erythema migrans.* The frequency with which such patients are seronegative, for whatever reason, suggests that serologic testing should not be done in patients with early Lyme disease. In fact, a negative test result in a patient with erythema migrans may dissuade from an appropriate clinical diagnosis. Although there are other skin lesions that mimic erythema migrans, if a patient with potential exposure to Lyme disease has a lesion suggesting erythema migrans, treatment, not testing, is suggested.

Some patients with early disseminated or early localized Lyme disease may still be seronegative if tested early enough in their disease. Patients with Lyme disease of longer duration—for example, 2 months or more—are very likely to be seropositive. Certainly patients with tertiary neuroborreliosis or Lyme arthritis are almost universally seropositive (1), and the diagnosis of late Lyme disease must be seriously questioned in patients who are seronegative.

Some clinicians who are fixated on the diagnosis of Lyme disease test repeatedly in patients who are seronegative in the hope of gaining serologic confirmation of the diagnosis. This represents a misuse of the laboratory testing. With the statistical methods used in ELISA, one is essentially assured that a positive test result will be obtained ultimately if the test is done often enough, and such a result would be a false-positive. In addition to wasting time, money, and effort, such a search usually also means that other, more likely causes of the patient's problem are not being investigated (see Case 10.2).

Effects of Antibiotic Therapy

Antibiotic treatment in early disease may abort seroconversion, even if the therapy is inadequate (13). Thus, if a patient receives a short course of antibiotics for a "summer cold" (e.g., erythromycin for 5 days)—therapy inadequate for the treatment of Lyme disease—or takes a few antibiotics left over from a previous prescription for an earlier infection, he or she may

---

CASE 10.2 *Early disseminated Lyme disease with mild neurologic manifestations*

A 33-year-old man presents with an expanding red rash on the left side of his groin. He noted a tick bite there 17 days ago and is now concerned that he might have Lyme disease. He has a moderate headache with a slight stiffness in his neck.

On examination, it is noted that there are an erythema migrans lesion on his groin that is 8 cm and three small, flat, asymptomatic erythematous lesions on his back that are 3 × 3 cm to 5 × 5 cm. The Kernig and Brudzinski signs are negative, but he has neck tenderness and moderate pain on neck flexion. Mild asymmetry of the face is noted, and a partial right seventh nerve palsy is identified.

Although the clinical findings indicate that the patient should be treated for Lyme disease at this visit, there are concerns that he might have central nervous system infection. A spinal tap produces clear fluid with 85 lymphocytes/mm^3 and an elevated protein level (87 mg/dL). Results of serum antibody testing reveal a negative IgG and IgM ELISA . Cerebrospinal fluid analysis reveals only IgM antibodies to the 41-kd antigen (flagellin). The negative result of serologic testing is interpreted as representing a test done too early in the course of the disease, and the IgM antibody to the 41-kd antigen is interpreted as a local intrathecal antibody response, confirming the diagnosis of Lyme meningitis. The patient receives intravenous ceftriaxone and responds well to this treatment over the next 8 days.

---

not have a sufficient antibody response to be detected in standard assays. The explanation for this phenomenon is not known, but the phenomenon may explain the *rare* example of a patient with later features of Lyme disease who is seronegative.

Concern about the effect of antibiotic therapy on testing results should not apply to patients with possible longstanding Lyme disease who have recently received antibiotics. Production of IgG in the response to *B. burgdorferi* does not stop immediately upon treatment with antibiotics. In fact, the immune response may persist for several weeks after termination of treatment. In any event, the half-life of serum IgG is approximately 22 days (4), so that antibody levels will persist (and therefore test results will remain positive) for a long time after treatment begins.

Interlaboratory Variation

Enzyme-linked immunosorbent assay and even Western blot results in different laboratories cannot be directly compared because of significant variation in reagents and techniques (14,15). In one study, identical serum samples were sent to different laboratories for ELISA testing; known positive sera were correctly identified in less than half of the cases, and there was nearly no agreement between the laboratories (14).

The laboratory provides the clinician with a standardized report for all patients, not an individualized interpretation for a *particular* patient. One must interpret results *in light of the clinical details* of that individual case, on information not available to the laboratory. Clinicians should find one laboratory that provides quality testing, that can provide more individualized clinical advice if given further information about the patient, and that is able to do more specialized testing if needed (such as the testing of inflammatory fluids).

Persistence of Seropositivity

High levels of IgG and occasionally of IgM may persist for several years after adequate treatment and resolution of symptoms (16,17). Persisting seropositivity is not diagnostic of ongoing infection, although it has often been misinterpreted as representing ongoing infection (18). For this reason, follow-up serologic testing in the patient who is asymptomatic or who is slowly improving should be discouraged (see Case 10.3).

The one circumstance in which follow-up serologic testing may be of value is the patient in whom the objective manifestations of Lyme disease are worsening or in whom new objective features of possible Lyme disease appear (e.g., a patient with erythema migrans who, months after appropriate treatment, develops monoarthritis). Of course, in such a setting one must consider an intercurrent illness as a cause of the current problem. However, if sequential studies demonstrate a rising ELISA titer and the appearance of new bands on Western blot (i.e., reactivity with proteins not previously recognized), the clinician must consider the possibility that this expanding immunologic repertoire reflects ongoing infection.

Nevertheless, one must be cautious in considering this possibility. Because antibody production does not abruptly halt when an antibiotic is given, new reactivity on Western blot may appear during the weeks that follow effective antibiotic therapy. An expanding immunologic repertoire does not indicate ongoing infection unless worsening or evolution of the clinical signs is also present.

Furthermore, comparison of test results cannot be made between different laboratories, and comparison between results obtained on different days in the same laboratory is problematic. Before one concludes that a significant change in the test results has occurred, one should consult with the laboratory staff to ensure that serologic reactivity has in fact changed. (The most accurate way of making such comparisons is with side-by-side testing of the serum samples that were taken on the different dates. Most commercial laboratories do not save serum samples, so such a comparison is usually not possible except at research laboratories.)

CASE 10.3.   *Irrelevant serologic reactivity*

Nine months ago, a 45-year-old man was diagnosed as having Lyme disease (he presented with erythema migrans and associated headache, which resolved during the 3-week course of treatment with doxycycline). He was seropositive at the time of the diagnosis but has decided to have a repeat serologic test done at the urging of a co-worker who is concerned that he might have "chronic Lyme disease." He is feeling well, with no new or specific symptoms. The results of his physical examination are normal.

Serologic testing 9 months ago revealed the following:

- Positive result for IgG and IgM on ELISA
- Immunoblot IgM reactivity with 23- and 41-kd bands
- Immunoblot IgG reactivity with 23-, 30-, 41-, 45-, 58-, 66-, and 93-kd bands
- Both IgM and IgG interpreted as positive

Current serologic testing reveals the following:

- Positive result for IgG and IgM on ELISA
- Immunoblot IgM reactivity with 23- and 41-kd bands
- Immunoblot IgG reactivity with 23-, 41-, and 93-kd bands
- IgM interpreted as positive

The clinical conclusion is that he has no evidence of active Lyme disease and that his persistent seropositivity is of no clinical significance.

Proper Use of Western Blot Criteria

As noted in Table 10.1, Western blot interpretation has two sets of criteria: one for early Lyme disease, which considers IgM reactivity; and a second for Lyme disease of longer duration, which is based on IgG reactivity. IgM reactivity may persist for many months or years, but in long-term infection, IgG reactivity appears uniformly. It is important not to apply the IgM criteria to patients with long-term symptoms who are being evaluated for late Lyme disease. Satisfaction of the IgM criteria suggests recent onset of disease; these criteria do not establish *active* or *ongoing* infection.

Studying Inflammatory Fluids

Patients with meningitis, encephalitis, and synovitis caused by *B. burgdorferi* will usually have local evidence of infection or immunologic reactivity to the organism (19,20). Although the organism has been identified in or grown from inflammatory fluid samples, such testing is not sufficiently sensitive or available to be of general clinical use.

In the proper clinical setting, testing of synovial or cerebrospinal fluids for the presence of specific antibodies to B. burgdorferi, especially for the presence of a relative concentration of antibodies in the inflammatory fluid compared with that found in the serum, is very useful in establishing the cause of the local inflammation. One can have serum antibodies to B. burgdorferi and still have another cause of seventh nerve palsy (e.g., Bell palsy), meningitis (e.g., enterovirus), headache (e.g., brain tumor), or monoarthritis (e.g., gout); seropositivity does not ensure that Lyme disease is the cause of the current inflammation.

Thus, one can measure antibodies in spinal or synovial fluid samples and compare the following:

- The levels of antibodies in the inflammatory fluid with those in serum, compensating for differences in albumin and total immunoglobulin. An elevated antibody level within the inflammatory fluid is strong evidence of local infection.
- Patterns of immunoblot reactivity. The finding of a "band" within the inflammatory fluid that is not present in serum or the presence of multiple IgM position bands within the thecal space in a minimally inflamed meninges is strong evidence of local infection.

Summary of the Usefulness of Serologic Tests

The presence of seroreactivity by ELISA and Western blot indicates the presence of antibodies to the organism that causes Lyme disease. It does not, however, make the diagnosis of Lyme disease, which should always be based on the clinical likelihood of the disease. Nor does seroreactivity establish the presence of active infection. As with all serologic tests, anti–B. burgdorferi antibody tests should be used only for confirmation of a clinical diagnosis. Positive and negative tests results have value in clinical decision-making when used in the right setting, taking into account the precautions noted earlier. For example,

- If the test is used in a population in which Lyme disease is very likely, such as in patients in an endemic area with isolated monoarthritis or bilateral facial nerve palsy, a positive test result is very likely to confirm the clinical suspicion that Lyme disease is present—that is, the test has a high positive-predictive value.
- In Lyme disease of long duration (e.g., tertiary neuroborreliosis or Lyme arthritis), seroreactivity by ELISA and Western blot is

nearly universal. Unless one can establish a reasonable cause, the absence of seroreactivity in such a patient should raise significant doubts about the diagnosis of Lyme disease—that is, the negative-predictive value of the test is very high.

- Seroreactivity may persist long after successful therapy has been given and the patient is cured (13). Persistence of seroreactivity is therefore not necessarily indicative of persisting infection in patients who have a long period of recovery (1,14).

- The presence of antibodies in the serum does not prove that the *current* clinical problems are caused by *B. burgdorferi*. When inflammatory joint disease or central nervous system disease is present, testing of the synovial or cerebrospinal fluid for the presence of *B. burgdorferi* antibodies and then comparing the results with the results of testing for the presence of these antibodies in the serum are invaluable in ensuring that the closed-space inflammation is caused by *B. burgdorferi* (15).

The term "Lyme disease test" should be abandoned: it is overly suggestive and easily misinterpreted as indicating that the positive test *makes* the diagnosis. Serologic tests are more accurately called "anti–*B. burgdorferi* antibody tests"—less euphonious, but a much more accurate term and one less prone to misuse. Finally, all tests are only as good as the clinician interpreting them.

Investigational Tests

Various assays have been proposed for use in confirming the diagnosis of Lyme disease (Box 10.1), but these tests have not been sufficiently studied to become a standard part of the Lyme disease armamentarium. All must be considered investigational, and their routine use in the clinical setting is not currently recommended.

Box 10.1   Investigational Lyme Disease Assays

Polymerase chain reaction
Urinary antigen testing
Borreliacidal antibody assay
Immune complex disruption
T-cell proliferative responses

Polymerase Chain Reaction

Polymerase chain reaction (PCR) is a very powerful technique that allows one to make millions of duplicate copies from a single copy of DNA in a biologic specimen (the term used is "to amplify" the DNA), enabling the identification of the genome of *B. burgdorferi* in cerebrospinal fluid, synovial fluid, or blood (21–26).

Preparation for PCR involves synthesizing a sequence of DNA known to be unique to the DNA of the intended target and not shared by other organisms; these synthesized sequences are called primers. The DNA from the specimen to be tested is isolated and added to a reaction mixture containing vast excesses of the primers and nucleotides that will become part of the synthesized DNA. Finally, an enzyme known as DNA polymerase is added, which can make the mirror-image match of DNA in the clinical sample.

DNA polymerase is active (i.e., DNA copying occurs) at a certain temperature. At higher temperatures, DNA denatures (the strands of DNA disassociate); when the reaction mixture is cooled, the target DNA and the primers reassociate ("reannealing"), and the enzyme makes a copy. By repeating this process, one can make large numbers of copies (repetition of the cycle 25 times produces 2^{25} copies of the DNA), which can be detected, whereas the original few copies could never have been identified.

The usefulness of PCR in the routine management of Lyme disease has not been verified, and its routine use cannot yet be advocated. Some of the limitations to the use and interpretation of PCR include the following (27):

- PCR is such a powerful tool, theoretically capable of identifying a single copy of *B. burgdorferi* DNA in a sample, that it is prone to false-positive results due to improper sample acquisition/handling or laboratory errors. Thus, the PCR result is only as useful as the care taken in obtaining the sample, and only as accurate as the care taken in the laboratory. PCR requires scrupulous care and appropriate controls at every step.

- Because *B. burgdorferi* is typically absent from blood samples of patients with late-stage Lyme disease, PCR is useful only in testing the inflammatory fluids (such as spinal and synovial fluids) of these patients.

- False-negative results can occur owing to the presence of biologic polymerase inhibitors in the specimen, including hemoglobin or hyaluronic acid.

- Polymerase chain reaction identifies DNA in the specimen, but it does not differentiate between live and dead organisms. Thus, PCR may be positive during active infection, in the presence of dead organisms, or in the presence of blebs liberated from an organism involved in previous, eradicated infection.

Urinary Antigen Testing

The urinary antigen test is based on the theory that as the organism grows in vivo, it sheds outer-surface proteins which may then be detected in urine or inflammatory fluids. The urine is concentrated and then filtered through a membrane which is subsequently probed for trapped urinary proteins with a monoclonal antibody. Other detection procedures have been used, as well.

Urine testing has been available for several years and has been the subject of several laboratory studies (28,29). It remains of unproven value. There is no evidence that it is more sensitive than the standard serologic tests. One unproven protocol is to use the assay both before and during the first few days of antibiotic therapy, in the belief that the organism liberates more antigen as it is killed. There is no current role for this test in the evaluation or management of patients with possible Lyme disease.

Borreliacidal Antibody Assay

The role of antibody in the immune response to infection is presumably to kill pathogens. Thus, a functional assay which measures in vitro killing of *Borrelia* might be effective in documenting exposure to *B. burgdorferi*. This assay (also known as the Gundersen Clinic assay) is commercially available (30,31). There are insufficient corroborative data from other laboratories to prove that it is as effective as or superior to other tests available.

Immune Complex Disruption

The fact that the results of standard ELISA are often negative in early disease is a major concern in the diagnosis of Lyme disease. One possible explanation for this phenomenon is that something about the organism delays the host's immune response. Alternatively, it may be that all antibodies bind to their intended targets shed by the organism, and the association of antibody with its target antigen forms an immune complex.

This hypothesis is supported by several observations:

- Immune complexes are found in the serum of patients with Lyme disease (32,33).
- Specific anti–*B. burgdorferi* antibody has been found in immune complexes in serum and cerebrospinal fluid samples (34–36).
- Certain borrelial proteins have been found in or associated with these immune complexes, and in some cases antibodies to borrelial proteins are found only in the complexes, not free in serum (37).

Testing for immune complexes is currently a laboratory tool with limited availability and unproven clinical value, although we believe such techniques hold very real promise (37).

T-Cell Proliferative Response

T cells that recognize borrelial antigens have been found in the blood, synovial fluid, and cerebrospinal fluid of patients with Lyme disease (38–42). Although T-cell testing is occasionally positive in the absence of serum antibodies (13), T-cell reactivity is more frequently accompanied by seroreactivity (43).

The consensus is that T-cell testing is not a promising confirmatory test for Lyme disease (11). Some reasons are as follows:

- T-cell testing is difficult to perform and interpret.
- Fresh T cells are required.
- The results are highly dependent on the preparation of *B. burgdorferi* that is being used.
- Interlaboratory variation is extreme, with some laboratories having many false-positive results and others having many false-negative results.

In some settings, however, this assay may be helpful, such as in testing inflammatory fluids (e.g., synovial and cerebrospinal fluids) (38,39). A local response—that is, concentration of immune reactivity within the closed-space with respect to the blood—confirms that the inflammation in these closed-spaces is related to local *B. burgdorferi* infection (19).

Cautions in the Use of Investigational Tests

The newer techniques await verification and standardization before they can be accepted for routine clinical use. Use of these tests is therefore currently discouraged. In cases in which there seems to be a need for more sophisticated testing to help confirm a diagnosis of Lyme disease, discussion or consultation with an academic center where clinical research is being done is warranted. In general, the standard tests in current use are sufficient to confirm the clinical diagnosis of Lyme disease.

Recommendations: The Use and Misuse of Tests

Lyme disease is a clinical diagnosis that can be confirmed by the judicious use of laboratory testing; diagnosis solely by serologic testing is a flawed process. In our experience, cases of Lyme disease that require use of the investigational tools or in which ELISA and Western blot are used repeatedly to confirm the diagnosis are usually not Lyme disease.

Use of the accepted serologic tests allows seroconfirmation of the diagnosis in most cases, although testing too early in the course of infection may lead to a false-negative result. Likewise, patients who receive antibiotic therapy very early in the course of their disease, even therapy inadequate to cure the infection, may be rendered seronegative despite having ongoing infection. Because of the problem with false-positive ELISA results, the adoption of the two-tier testing strategy—ELISA (if positive) followed by Western blot—is advocated.

Comparison of antibody levels (by ELISA) and specificities (by immunoblot) in both inflammatory fluid and serum is an invaluable tool to ensure that the close-space inflammatory condition is in fact caused by Lyme disease and not by an intercurrent extraneous medical problem. Finally, new techniques and new antigenic preparations (e.g., using recombinant proteins or peptide epitopes rather than a crude sonicate of *B. burgdorferi*) may lead to more accurate and useful methods of confirming the clinical diagnosis of Lyme disease.

■ ■ ■

Key Points

- The diagnosis of Lyme disease is based solely on objective clinical findings, with serologic test results used only to confirm the diagnosis. Serologic tests are not "diagnostic tests": They are "confirmatory tests."

- IgM is the predominant antibody early in the primary immune response; IgG is the predominant class later in the primary response and in the secondary immune response. IgM positivity is *not* equivalent to active infection.

- All positive or equivocal ELISA results must be confirmed by immunoblot analysis owing to the high frequency of false-positive results with ELISA.

- Urine antigen testing and T-cell proliferation assays have no defined role in the diagnosis or management of Lyme disease.

- Polymerase chain reaction remains an experimental tool and should not be used in patient management decisions; PCR does not differentiate between live and dead organisms.

■ ■ ■

REFERENCES

1. **Steere AC.** Lyme disease. N Engl J Med. 1989;321:586-96.

2. **Pachner AR.** *Borrelia burgdorferi* in the nervous system: the new "Great Imitator." Ann N Y Acad Sci. 1988;539:56-64.

3. **Finkel MJ, Halperin JJ.** Nervous system Lyme borreliosis—revisited. Arch Neurol. 1992;49:102-7.

4. **Sigal LH, Plescia O.** Antibodies: structure and function. In: Sigal LH, Ron Y, eds. Immunology and inflammation: basic mechanisms and clinical consequences. New York: McGraw-Hill; 1993: 37-62.

5. **Weiss NL, Sadock VA, Sigal LH, et al.** False positive seroreactivity to *Borrelia burgdorferi* in systemic lupus erythematosus: the value of immunoblot analysis. Lupus. 1995;4:131-7.

6. **Magnarelli LA, Miller JN, Anderson JF, Riviere GR.** Cross-reactivity of nonspecific treponemal antibody in serologic tests for Lyme disease. J Clin Microbiol. 1990;28:1276-9.

7. **Magnarelli LA, Anderson JF.** Enzyme-linked immunosorbent assays for the detection of class-specific immunoglobulins to *Borrelia burgdorferi*. Am J Epidemiol. 1988;127:818-25.

8. **Kaell AT, Redecha PR, Elkon KB, et al.** Occurrence of antibodies to *Borrelia burgdorferi* in patients with nonspirochetal subacute bacterial endocarditis. Ann Intern Med. 1993;119:1079-83.

9. **Dressler F, Whalen JA, Reinhardt BN, Steere AC.** Western blotting in the serodiagnosis of Lyme disease. J. Infect Dis. 1993;167:392-400.

10. **Centers for Disease Control and Prevention.** Recommendations for test performance from the Second National Conference on Serologic Diagnosis of Lyme Disease. MMWR Morb Mortal Wkly Rep. 1995;44:590-1.

11. **Sigal LH.** Lyme disease: a review of aspects of its immunology and immunopathogenesis. Annu Rev Immunol. 1997;15:63-92.

12. **Lightfoot RW Jr, Luft BJ, Rahn DW, et al.** Empiric parenteral antibiotic treatment of patients with fibromyalgia and fatigue and a positive result for Lyme disease: a cost-effectiveness analysis. Ann Intern Med. 1993;119:503-9.

13. **Dattwyler RJ, Volkman DJ, Luft BJ, et al.** Seronegative Lyme disease: dissociation of specific T- and B-lymphocyte responses to *B. burgdorferi*. N Engl J Med. 1988;319:1441-6.

14. **Bakken LL, Case KL, Callister SM, et al.** Performance of 45 laboratories participating in a proficiency testing program for Lyme disease serology. JAMA. 1992;268:891-6.

15. **Craven RB, Quan T, Bailey RE, et al.** Improved serodiagnostic testing for Lyme disease: results of a multicenter serologic evaluation. Emerg Infect Dis. 1996;2:136-40.

16. **Feder HM Jr, Gerber MA, Luger SW, Ryan RW.** Persistence of serum antibodies to *Borrelia burgdorferi* in patients treated for Lyme disease. Clin Infect Dis. 1992;15:788-92.

17. **Hilton E, Tramontano A, DeVoti J, Sood SK.** Temporal study of immunoglobulin M seroreactivity to *Borrelia burgdorferi* in patients treated for Lyme borreliosis. J Clin Microbiol. 1997;35:774-6.

18. **Sigal LH.** Persisting complaints attributed to Lyme disease: possible mechanisms and implications for management. Am J Med. 1994;96:365-75.

19. **Steere AC, Berardi VP, Weeks KE, et al.** Evaluation of the intrathecal antibody response to *Borrelia burgdorferi* as a diagnostic test for Lyme neuroborreliosis. J Infect Dis. 1990; 161:1203-9.

20. **Sigal LH.** *B. burgdorferi (BB)*-specific immune reactivity (IR) at the site of Lyme disease (LD) inflammation. Presented at the IV International Conference on Lyme Borreliosis, Stockholm, Sweden, June 18–21, 1990. Stockholm, Sweden: Almqvist & Wiksell International; 1991.

21. **Liebling MR, Nishio MJ, Rodriguez A, et al.** The polymerase chain reaction for the detection of *Borrelia burgdorferi* in human body fluids. Identification of *Borrelia burgdorferi* using interrupted polymerase chain reaction. Arthritis Rheum. 1993;36:665-75.

22. **Nocton JJ, Dressler F, Rutledge BJ, et al.** Detection of *Borrelia burgdorferi* DNA by polymerase chain reaction in synovial fluid from patients with Lyme arthritis. N Engl J Med. 1994;330:229-34.

23. **Keller TL, Halperin JJ, Whitman M.** PCR detection of *Borrelia burgdorferi* DNA in cerebrospinal fluid of Lyme neuroborreliosis patients. Neurology. 1992;42:32-42.

24. **Schwartz I, Wormser GP, Schwartz JJ, et al.** Diagnosis of early Lyme disease by polymerase chain reaction amplification and culture of skin biopsies from erythema migrans lesions. J Clin Microbiol. 1992;30:3082-8.

25. **Pachner AR, Delaney E.** The polymerase chain reaction (PCR) in the diagnosis of Lyme neuroborreliosis. Ann Neurol. 1993;34:544-50.

26. **Bradley JF, Johnson RC, Goodman JL.** The persistence of spirochetal nucleic acids in active Lyme arthritis. Ann Intern Med. 1994;120:487-9

27. **Sigal LH.** The polymerase chain reaction assay for *Borrelia burgdorferi* in the diagnosis of Lyme disease [editorial]. Ann Intern Med. 1994;120:520-1.

28. **Dorwood DW, Schwan TG, Garon CF.** Immune capture and detection of *Borrelia burgdorferi* antigens in urine, blood, or tissues from infected ticks, mice, dogs, and humans. J Clin Microbiol. 1991;29:1162-70.

29. **Magnarelli LA, Anderson JF, Stafford KC III.** Detection of *Borrelia burgdorferi* in urine of *Permyscus leucopus* by inhibition enzyme-linked immunosorbent assay. J Clin Microbiol. 1994;32:777-82.

30. **Callister SM, Schell RL, Case KL, et al.** Characterization of the borreliacidal antibody response to *Borrelia burgdorferi* in humans: a serodiagnostic test. J Infect Dis. 1993; 167:158-64.

31. **Callister SM, Schell RF, Lim LC, et al.** Detection of borreliacidal antibodies by flow cytometry: an accurate, highly specific serodiagnostic test for Lyme disease. Arch Intern Med. 1994;154:1625-32.

32. **Hardin JA, Walker LC, Steere AC, et al.** Circulating immune complexes in Lyme arthritis: detection by the ^{125}I-C1q binding, C1q solid phase, and Raji cell assays. J Clin Invest. 1979;63:468-77.

33. **Hardin JA, Steere AC, Malawista SE.** Immune complexes and the evolution of Lyme arthritis: dissemination and localization of abnormal C1q binding activity. N Engl J Med. 1979; 301:1358-63.

34. **Schutzer SE, Coyle PK, Dunn JJ, et al.** Early and specific antibody response to OspA in Lyme disease. J Clin Invest. 1994;94:454-7

35. **Coyle PK, Schutzer SE, Belman AL, et al.** Cerebrospinal fluid immune complexes in patients exposed to *Borrelia burgdorferi*: detection of Borrelia-specific and nonspecific complexes. Ann Neurol. 1990;28:739-44.

36. **Schutzer SE, Coyle PK, Belman AL, et al.** Sequestration of antibody to *Borrelia burgdorferi* in immune complexes in seronegative Lyme disease. Lancet. 1990;335:312-5.

37. **Brunner M, Stein S, Sigal LH.** Enzyme-linked IgM capture immune complex biotinylated-antigen assay (EMIBA): A new immunoassay for early Lyme disease. Arthritis Rheum. 1997;40:1645.

38. **Sigal LH, Steere AC, Freeman DH, Dwyer JM.** Proliferative responses of mononuclear cells in Lyme disease: concentration of *Borrelia burgdorferi*–reactive cells in joint fluid. Arthritis Rheum. 1986;29:761-9.

39. **Pachner AR, Steere AC, Sigal LH, Johnson CJ.** Antigen-specific proliferation of CSF lymphocytes in Lyme disease. Neurology. 1985;35:1642-44.

40. **Dressler F, Yoshinari NH, Steere AC.** The T-cell proliferative assay in the diagnosis of Lyme disease. Ann Intern Med. 1991;115:533-40.

41. **Krause A, Burmester GR, Rensing A, et al.** Cellular immune reactivity to recombinant OspA and flagellin from *Borrelia burgdorferi* in patients with Lyme borreliosis. J Clin Invest. 1992;90:1077-84.

42. **Zoschke DC, Skemp AA, Defosse DL.** Lymphoproliferative responses to *Borrelia burgdorferi* in Lyme disease. Ann Intern Med. 1991;114:285-9.

43. **Sigal LH.** Utility of T cell anti-*B. burgdorferi* reactivity (T-BB) in diagnosing Lyme disease (LD). Presented at the IV International Conference on Lyme Borreliosis, Stockholm, Sweden. June 18-21, 1990. Stockholm, Sweden: Almqvist & Wiksell International; 1991.

KEY REFERENCES

Bradley JF, Johnson RC, Goodman JL. The persistence of spirochetal nucleic acids in active Lyme arthritis. Ann Intern Med. 1994;120:487-9.

Kaell AT, Redecha PR, Elkon KB, et al. Occurrence of antibodies to *Borrelia burgdorferi* in patients with nonspirochetal subacute bacterial endocarditis. Ann Intern Med. 1993;119:1079-83.

*Describes other diseases in which false-positive ELISA results may be obtained. Eloquent reasons for abandoning the term "Lyme disease test" in favor of the more correct (and less suggestive) "anti-*Borrelia burgdorferi *antibody assay."*

Sigal LH. The polymerase chain reaction assay for *Borrelia burgdorferi* in the diagnosis of Lyme disease [editorial]. Ann Intern Med. 1994;120:520-1.

Discusses how PCR is a valuable research tool, but it is premature to use it as a diagnostic test. PCR does not differentiate between living and dead organisms and therefore cannot establish active infection from the persistence of dead organisms.

Sigal LH. Lyme disease: a review of aspects of its immunology and immunopathogenesis. Annu Rev Immunol. 1997;15:63-92.

*Summary of the current understanding of the human immune and inflammatory response to *Borrelia burgdorferi *infection.*

Sigal LH. Pitfalls in the diagnosis and management of Lyme disease: Special article. Arthritis Rheum. 1997 [In press].

A review of many of the uses and misuses of testing, especially in the management of patients with prior evidence of B. burgdorferi infection. More detailed discussion of the positive and negative predictive values (PPV and NPV) of serologic testing.

Steere AC, Berardi VP, Weeks KE, et al. Evaluation of the intrathecal antibody response to *Borrelia burgdorferi* as a diagnostic test for Lyme neuroborreliosis. J Infect Dis. 1990;161:1203-9.

An important discussion of the value of looking for locally produced immune reactivity—in this case, antibodies within the thecal space—but the same is true within the synovial cavity and for T-cell reactivity as well.

Weiss NL, Sadock VA, Sigal LH, et al. False positive seroreactivity to *B. burgdorferi* in systemic lupus erythematosus: the value of immunoblot analysis. Lupus. 1995;4:131-7.

Immunoblot is useful in inflammatory disease to identify ELISA reactivity as a false-positive test in systemic lupus erythematosus and rheumatoid arthritis.

11

■ ■ ■

Disease Management in Lyme Disease: From Consensus to Care

Anthony D. So, MD, MPA

Daniel W. Rahn, MD

mproving the diagnosis and management of Lyme disease is a challenge. Although various guidelines have been promulgated, a gap remains between the *recommended* approach to diagnosis and treatment and the approaches that are actually most commonly used in clinical practice.

Many barriers interfere with the acceptance of evidence-based recommendations as guidelines for routine clinical care for patients with suspected Lyme disease. Some obstacles are difficult to quantify and involve issues such as physician diagnostic uncertainty and patient expectations regarding testing or treatment. Understanding these factors may allow us to develop a disease management program that has a higher likelihood of acceptance in clinical practice.

In this chapter, we examine the essential components of a comprehensive disease management program for Lyme disease and some of the barriers to eliminating practice variations. With support from the Centers for Disease Control and Prevention (CDC), the American College of Physicians has developed a disease management program for Lyme disease that takes these issues into consideration. This program should have broad applicability to physician practice and to health plans attempting to design disease management systems and to adapt guidelines to local use.

Physician Adoption of Practice Guidelines

Several efforts have been undertaken to develop guidelines for the diagnosis and treatment of Lyme disease. Professional societies, such as the American College of Physicians' Clinical Efficacy Assessment Program (CEAP), and expert groups convened by CDC and the National Institutes of Health (NIH) have deliberated and released practice guidelines (1–6). In the peer-reviewed literature, experts in Lyme disease have also advanced their own recommendations for evaluation and management (6-8).

These guideline efforts provide a framework for physician decision making. However, clinician confidence in practice guidelines depends on several factors. In a survey of members of the American College of Physicians, respondents reported greater confidence in guidelines issued by specialty organizations rather than those by the American Medical Association or certain federal agencies (9). Internists working on a fixed salary, those working fewer than 20 hours per week, or those not in private practice held more favorable attitudes towards guidelines.

While usually evidence based, guidelines often do not adequately consider the motivations behind physician practice and thus may have a less-than-desirable impact on clinical decision making. To move from consensus to care, the gulf between guidelines and practice must be narrowed by considering these motivations. Endemicity and the familiarity of clinicians with the disease likely influence the threshold to test, to treat, and to refer. Concern over potential adverse outcomes can influence how a physician responds to uncertainty. Symptoms that do not fully resolve may be interpreted as treatment failure rather than as unrealistic expectations or misdiagnosis. And patient pressure for diagnostic evaluation may lead to inappropriate use of laboratory tests.

These factors and others play out differently in different local practice settings and must be considered in designing disease management programs intended for broad implementation. Physicians may be slow to accept guidelines for the management of Lyme disease because of errors in diagnosis, inadequate appreciation of the true magnitude of disease risk, and the difficulties associated with meeting unrealistic patient expectations that are often grounded in misinformation.

Factors Contributing to Errors in Diagnosis

Although cases of Lyme disease are being recognized more often than in the past, several studies indicate that misdiagnosis is quite common. In fact, in some studies, misdiagnosis was more common than correct diagnosis. Steere and colleagues (10) reported that 57% of 788 patients referred to a university Lyme disease clinic over a 4.5-year period did *not* have the disease. Of the referred patients without Lyme disease, 45% had previously tested positive in serologic tests for Lyme disease, but repeat testing at the university clinic was negative. Of those who previously received treatment with antibiotics, nearly four out of five failed to respond to therapy because of incorrect diagnosis.

A study at another university Lyme disease clinic characterized problems of overdiagnosis and underdiagnosis among pediatric patients (11). Only half were correctly diagnosed. The errors ranged from misdiagnosing rashes as erythema migrans and nonspecific symptoms as Lyme disease, to failing to diagnose fleeting objective symptoms of Lyme disease.

Several factors have been identified that contribute to clinician uncertainty in diagnosing Lyme disease (Box 11.1).

Clinicians struggle with the diagnosis of Lyme disease because it is perceived to have protean manifestations. Particularly in nonendemic areas, clinicians may not have had the experience of making the diagnosis of typical early Lyme disease—namely, diagnosis based on recognition of erythema migrans. Resorting to serologic testing can produce false-positive results and thus creates a false impression of what the clinical spectrum of Lyme disease actually is. For these physicians, treatment of patients with atypical clinical syndromes becomes anchored on false-positive test results.

Competing diagnoses also complicate the evaluation of Lyme disease. Notably, in the southeastern United States, an erythema migrans–like disease caused by a tick-transmitted agent other than *Borrelia burgdorferi* is being increasingly recognized (12,12A). The natural history of this disorder and its response to therapy differ from those of Lyme disease.

The clinician must also distinguish chronic Lyme disease from fibromyalgia and chronic fatigue syndrome, the most common competing diagnoses (13). Both of these disorders carry uncertain prognoses, with most patients having chronic, persistent symptoms and for which there is no "magic bullet" resolution. Patients are understandably reluctant to accept these diagnoses and thus exert pressure on their physicians to search for alternative diagnoses. Although Lyme disease may trigger fibromyalgia,

---

Box 11.1   Factors Contributing to Uncertainty in Diagnosing Lyme Disease

Protean manifestations
Competing diagnoses
Inappropriate use and interpretation of serologic tests
Absence of a "gold standard" diagnostic test or feature
Difficulty in understanding local endemicity

treatment with antibiotics has not proved to be effective in resolving the symptoms and signs of fibromyalgia (14). Serologic tests are often ordered in patients with fibromyalgia in the hope that Lyme disease may be found, since this condition *does* respond to definitive, antibiotic therapy. However, whether patients are seropositive in Lyme disease testing is irrelevant to the diagnosis and management of fibromyalgia.

It is easy to understand how resolving the uncertainty of protean manifestations and competing diagnoses often leads clinicians to the use of serologic testing. A true-positive serologic test result indicates exposure to, but not active infection with, *Borrelia burgdorferi*. The predictive value of a positive serologic test result (i.e., the probability that a person with a positive serologic test result actually has the disease) hinges on the pre-test probability of the presence of the disease. In many clinical settings, the pre-test probability is not known, because the clinician may not know the local endemicity or seroprevalence of Lyme disease. In nonendemic areas, clinicians may have limited experience in making the bedside diagnosis. As a result, it may not be possible to know with certainty the predictive value of a positive serologic test result.

In sum, these problems reveal that in common clinical practice, no single gold standard reference exists for the diagnosis of Lyme disease. Only culture-confirmed cases can represent such a standard. The CDC has undertaken developing a reference case series based on culture-confirmed Lyme disease, which may be the most important initiative in addressing this source of uncertainty.

In the meantime, a Lyme disease management program must account for these sources of clinician uncertainty. There is a difference between the appropriate threshold for treatment and the criteria for definitive diagnosis. Clinicians need guidance in how best to proceed when the diagnosis is uncertain. Without eliminating all uncertainty, simple physician and patient educational interventions can improve the diagnosis of Lyme disease (Box 11.2).

Box 11.2   Educational Building Blocks to an Effective Disease Management Program

Tick identification
Skin lesion recognition
Proper use of diagnostic tests
Expected clinical response to treatment
Endemicity in local geographic regions

Gauging the Probability of Disease

When a patient presents with an erythematous skin rash and a history of tick exposure, how do physicians assess the pre-test probability of Lyme disease? Many clinical clues, from duration of tick attachment to the season of the year, enter into this estimation. Both local disease prevalence and the presence (or absence) of characteristic clinical findings figure into the pre-test probability of Lyme disease. By proper use of these epidemiologic and clinical data, physicians can reduce or avoid unnecessary diagnostic testing.

Pre-test and Post-test Probabilities in Serologic Testing

Figure 11.1 shows the diagnostic yield, or post-test probability, after sero-logic testing in patients at various levels of pre-test probability of disease. When applied to the same spectrum of disease, each diagnostic test pos-sesses a sensitivity and specificity that do not vary. Regardless of the diag-nostic test characteristics (e.g., a test with a sensitivity of 95% and a specificity of 95% versus a test with a sensitivity of 75% and a specificity of 85%), the post-test probability depends on pre-test probability.

When the pre-test probability is very low or very high, the serologic test does little to improve diagnostic certainty. When the pre-test probabil-ity starts low, the post-test probability remains low, and the treatment deci-sion therefore remains unchanged. Similarly, when the pre-test probability starts high, the post-test probability remains high when the test result is positive—and again, the treatment decision remains unchanged.

However, when the pre-test probability is in the range of 40% to 60%, the diagnostic test results can significantly change the post-test probability of disease. Similarly, if the pre-test probability is high, but the test result is negative, the post-test probability may be substantially lower. In both cases, the use of serologic testing can shift the treatment decision.

Likelihood Ratio

The actual contribution of a diagnostic test result can be quantified mathe-matically with use of a likelihood ratio. By definition, the likelihood ratio is the ratio of the probability of a positive test result in patients with Lyme disease to the probability of a positive test result in patients without the disease [i.e., sensitivity/(1 − specificity)] (15). Like sensitivity and specificity, the likelihood ratio itself is a characteristic of the test and is independent of pre-test probability or disease prevalence. For a positive serologic test re-sult for Lyme disease, the likelihood ratio has been estimated to be 5.0. When the serologic test is negative, the likelihood ratio is 0.06. In Figure 11.2, a nomogram maps this relationship between pre-test and post-test probability.

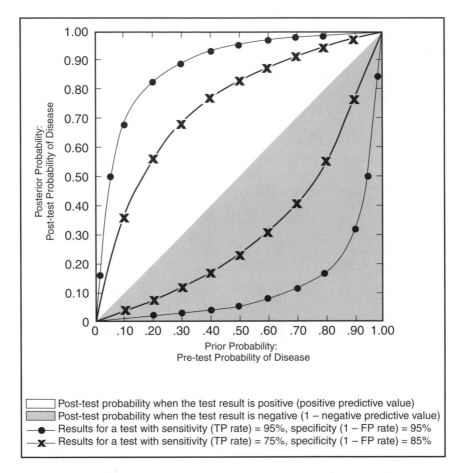

Figure 11.1 Post-test probability of disease after serologic testing according to pre-test probability. TP = true positive; FP = false positive. (Reprinted with permission from Sackett DL, Haynes RB, Guyatt GH, Tugwell P. *Clinical Epidemiology: A Basic Science for Clinical Medicine*. 2nd ed. Boston: Little, Brown & Co., 1991.)

The Decision to Treat

Whereas statistical information informs clinical judgment, the threshold to treat depends on other concerns as well. Even with a post-test probability of only 6%, as in the previous example, the decision may still be that a therapeutic trial is necessary. For example, patient preference or physician concern about the consequences of not treating 1 patient in 20 may outweigh considerations regarding the minimal risks of adverse drug reaction.

On the other hand, the possibility that the disease is most likely not Lyme disease must also be considered. In some areas endemic for Lyme

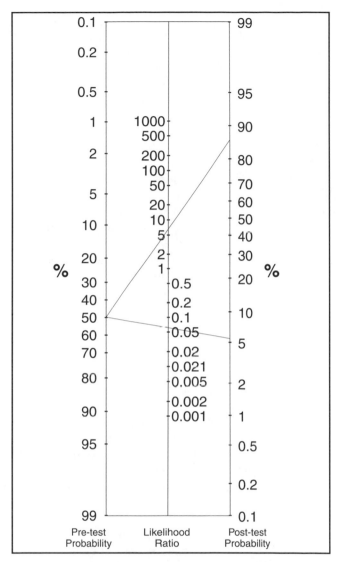

Figure 11.2   Nomogram for interpreting the relationship between pre-test and post-test probability. By drawing a line from the pre-test probability through the likelihood ratio of 5.0, one can find the post-test probability from a positive test result. For an individual with an estimated pre-test probability of Lyme disease of 50%, the post-test probability is increased to 86% if the serology is positive. When the serologic test is negative (likelihood ratio of 0.06), the post-test probability in the same patient drops to 6%. (Modified with permission from Tugwell P, Dennis DT, Weinstein A, et al. Laboratory evaluation in the diagnosis of Lyme disease. Clinical Guideline, Part 2. Ann Intern Med. 1997;127:1109-23.

disease, *Ixodes scapularis*, the tick vector for Lyme disease, also carries the agent for human granulocytic ehrlichiosis (HGE) (16). The local emergence of HGE may prompt the clinician to reconsider the risks and benefits of prescribing prophylactic antibiotic treatment to a person who has received a tick bite. Because the downhill course of HGE can be rapid, sometimes fatal, and without telltale rash, clinicians may find the risks of not prescribing *prophylactic* antibiotic treatment to a person with a tick bite greater than if only Lyme disease (which has a longer incubation period, often a telltale rash, and little risk of fatality) were on the differential diagnosis. To further complicate matters, although only doxycycline (and not amoxicillin) provides the reassurance of prophylactic coverage for both Lyme disease and HGE, particularly in pediatric cases, amoxicillin may be perferred over doxycycline for the treatment of Lyme disease. In any event, what is critically important is recognizing that when the diagnosis is unlikely to be Lyme disease, treatment for Lyme disease may not affect the disease course. In such cases, the search for other, perhaps more likely, causes must not be abandoned even if the decision is made to administer a therapeutic trial of antibiotics for possible Lyme disease.

Patient Expectations

Patient expectations may also influence a physician's decision to perform a diagnostic test or to institute empiric therapy. In a prepaid health plan in northern California, a study of patients tested for Lyme disease revealed that the patients themselves prompted serologic testing in 35% of cases (17). In only 19% of cases was the serologic test performed because the physician actually suspected Lyme disease.

When a patient has nonspecific complaints and a possible history of tick exposure, the level of clinical suspicion of Lyme disease is low. Serologic testing is more likely to produce a false-positive result, and as a result, inappropriate treatment is more likely to be given. This is particularly problematic in persons with fibromyalgia or with ill-defined neurologic syndromes. Therapy may begin with a false-positive serologic test and then continue based on an incomplete response or absence of well-defined endpoints to the therapeutic trial.

When patient expectations drive decision making, disease management must involve a prominent component of patient education. The public needs a more accurate understanding of disease risk and disease course as well as of expected response to therapy. Education tools, such as pamphlets, videotapes, or even interactive shared decision-making programs, can assist the physician in patient education.

ACP Disease Management Program for Lyme Disease

To accomplish its intended purpose, a disease management program for Lyme disease must account for the issues already discussed in this chapter—and yet others that also influence physician practice and narrow practice variation. These include education, feedback, physician participation, administrative rules, and financial incentives and penalties (18). These factors may change the threshold at which physicians refer for consultation, a major decision point in disease management.

Local factors play a role. When filing case report forms is easy or difficult, cases may go over- or under-reported. In turn, local estimates of disease prevalence may be affected, and these estimates may impact on local physicians' thresholds for diagnosing Lyme disease. In Georgia, hundreds of Lyme disease cases were reported until a survey of ticks revealed that few ticks in that region carried the spirochete (19).

Despite a common base of knowledge, variations in practice may still persist. In studies of small geographic areas in New England, Wennberg and colleagues discovered significant practice variations—fourfold differences in hysterectomy and prostatectomy rates (20,21). These were not explained by clinical, epidemiologic, or socioeconomic differences in the populations. Rather, they appeared to represent differences in the epidemiology of practice, not the epidemiology of disease. In an effort to address unexplained practice variation, the Maine Medical Assessment Foundation has organized specialty study groups to examine variations in local practice patterns. A study group on hospitalization for orthopedic conditions used utilization data as background for discussion of clinical issues and areas of uncertainty. Where peer group consensus did not support high rates of procedures, practice patterns have changed and rates reportedly have dropped, thus reducing practice variation (22). Use of feedback from administrative data on discharge rates is central to this effort. Although promising, this approach is labor intensive and best suited to expensive procedures.

Evaluation of clinical performance, however, does not follow easily from administrative data in many circumstances, particularly those not involving hospitalization or specific procedures. As in Lyme disease, case identification poses a significant challenge for clinicians, and in this regard, administrative data are of little assistance. In primary care medicine, many clinical decisions do not lend themselves easily to administrative data capture. Procedures do not figure prominently in the evaluation and treatment decisions in Lyme disease, so again, administrative data are often not helpful in monitoring these clinical practices.

An effective disease management program for Lyme disease must be based on approaches other than simple dissemination of practice guidelines, administrative data capture, and administrative rules. As a professional society, the American College of Physicians embarked on development of a Lyme disease management program that tapped other approaches—education, feedback, and physician participation. To accomplish these aims, the ACP applied lessons learned from health services research to continuing medical education (CME).

With the support of the Centers for Disease Control, the ACP Initiative on Lyme Disease uses a case-based format to deliver a CME program. CME is the usual means of providing ongoing education to physicians in practice and enabling them to keep their knowledge current. Generally delivered through rounds or clinical conferences, physicians learn clinical reasoning through case examples (23). The use of these clinical vignettes centers the teaching around cases that many physicians do not have the opportunity to see firsthand. Lyme disease is particularly well suited to case-based learning because the disease incidence is low in many areas, yet it surfaces on the differential diagnosis list quite often. In fact, its later manifestations are unfamiliar to many practicing physicians.

Case-Based Learning System

To these ends, the American College of Physicians has developed a program to teach through a case-based approach. With the input of an expert advisory committee, pivotal clinical cues and conundrums in the physician's decision-making process were identified. Next, clinical vignettes were constructed to illustrate these points, and storyboards were created. A videotape was prepared of carefully constructed, illustrative doctor–patient encounters, with expert narration that explains the decision-making following each clinical vignette.

Before the expert narrates each case, however, an audience-response system presents a series of key questions on Lyme disease and clinical decision making. Through the use of hand-held keypads, physicians record their answers to the questions posed about the clinical vignettes. Their answers are displayed graphically in aggregate to the entire group (although the answers of the individual physicians remain anonymous). When there is one answer that reflects the expert consensus, it is highlighted among the options. This interactive feedback can motivate the individual respondent, who sees his or her response against the background of peer and expert norms. Using this approach, the disease management program telescopes community practice variations into a classroom.

The videotaped expert narration explains the decision making in each case. However, an on-site facilitator—sometimes a local opinion leader—can walk through the questions and discuss clinical points in greater detail. This facilitator is particularly helpful when community and expert norms diverge or when the physician audience is sharply divided in their responses.

This approach pulls together the findings of community practice variations, the consensus of experts, and evidence-based guidelines and provides immediate feedback on where they differ. Typically, monitoring community-based practice variations requires access to administrative or other health care utilization data. Using standard cases on videotape ensures that each physician responds to the same stimuli, and differences among individual practices are then presented graphically. The discussion shifts from how practices and patients differ to why clinical decision making differs and is based on clinical issues, not administrative feedback. Recommendations of clinical guidelines and expert panel consensus can be highlighted by the facilitator/discussant, who is armed with the knowledge of how these mirror or differ from the current practices of the physicians in attendance.

The clinical vignettes can give structure to the discussion of clinical pathways. In doing so, this program can also facilitate the local adaptation of national guidelines. By studying practice demographics and clinical decisions, we can learn about the threshold for subspecialist referral, the office use of procedures such as lumbar puncture, or how firsthand experience with Lyme disease affects clinical decision making. As the program travels from community to community, it can evolve to focus on sources of clinical uncertainty or disagreement discovered along the way and stored in the audience response system database.

Continuing medical education interventions that use practice-enabling or reinforcing strategies consistently lead to improved physician performance (24). During the program on Lyme disease, the audience response system provides a measure of reinforcement as answers are reflected back to participants. In addition, the videotape introduces clinical practice tools, such as the nomogram, guidelines for diagnostic testing and treatment, and photographs to assist in identifying skin lesions and ticks, components that are intended to provide practice support for clinicians.

On the practice-enabling side, a final component of the American College of Physicians Disease Management Program includes patient education tools. The physician's decision not to test or treat will not allay patient anxiety and may only heighten patient pressure. Direct patient education materials have been developed to supplement the physician visit and reinforce the rationale for diagnostic and treatment decisions.

Conclusion

Nationwide, efforts are well under way to limit practice variation, reduce unnecessary health care expenditures, and measure and improve patient outcomes. In order to be successful, a disease management program must address the full array of issues that affect decision-making by both patients and clinicians. Ideally, such a program would incorporate perspectives from all "stakeholders," including physician experts, professional societies, public health entities, local providers, patients, payers, and health plans. It also must recognize the realities of clinical practice: evidence from peer-reviewed literature may only tell part of the story with regard to best practice. Sometimes clinical decision making in the office may appropriately differ from what a professional society would conclude is best practice based on evidence alone.

To bridge this gulf between expert consensus and local care, the disease management program developed by the American College of Physicians recognizes this dichotomy through presentations of both clinical evidence and case discussions. Through this work, the program hopes to strike a balance that optimizes patient outcomes and provides a framework for continuous quality improvement.

Acknowledgment.   This publication was supported in part by cooperative agreement number U50/CCU310312 from the Centers for Disease Control and Prevention (CDC). Its contents are solely the responsibility of the authors and the views expressed in this article do not necessarily represent the official views of the Agency for Health Care Policy and Research, the CDC, and/or the Department of Health and Human Services.

■   ■   ■

Key Points

- Factors such as competing diagnoses, the absence of a gold standard, and inappropriate use and interpretation of serologic tests contribute to clinician uncertainty in diagnosing Lyme disease.

- Patient expectations may influence physician decisions to perform diagnostic tests or institute empiric therapy.

- Patient education, including pamphlets and interactive media, can help address and sometimes modify these expectations.

- To gain acceptance in practice, a Lyme disease management program must encompass current community practice, the consensus of experts, and best evidence in the formulation of clinical pathways.

■   ■   ■

REFERENCES

1. NIH State-of-the-Art Conference. Diagnosis and Treatment of Lyme Disease. Clinical Courier. 1991;9:1–8.

2. Consensus Conference on Lyme Disease. Can Med Assoc J. 1991;144:1627–32.

3. Appropriateness of Parenteral Antibiotic Treatment for Patients with Presumed Lyme Disease: A Joint Statement of the American College of Rheumatology and the Council of the Infectious Diseases Society of America. Ann Intern Med. 1993; 119:518.

4. **Tugwell P, Dennis DT, Weinstein A, et al.** Laboratory evaluation in the diagnosis of Lyme disease. Clinical Guideline, Part 2. Ann Intern Med. 1997;127:1109-23.

5. Treatment of Lyme Disease. Med Lett Drugs Ther. 1992;39:47–8.

6. **Halperin JJ, Logigian EL, Finkel MF, Pearl RA.** Practice parameters for the diagnosis of patients with nervous system Lyme borreliosis (Lyme disease). Neurology. 1996;46:619–27.

7. **Rahn DW, Malawista SE.** Lyme disease: recommendations for diagnosis and treatment. Ann Intern Med. 1991;114:472–81.

8. **Steere AC.** Lyme Disease. N Engl J Med. 1989;321:586–96.

9. **Tunis SR, Hayward RS, Wilson MC, et al.** Internists' attitudes about clinical practice guidelines. Ann Intern Med. 1994;120:956–63.

10. **Steere AC, Taylor E, McHugh GL, Logigian EL.** The overdiagnosis of Lyme disease. JAMA. 1993;269:1812–16.

11. **Feder HM Jr, Hunt MS.** Pitfalls in the diagnosis and treatment of Lyme disease in children. JAMA. 1995;274:66–8.

12. **Campbell GS, Paul WS, Schriefer ME, et al.** Epidemiologic and diagnostic studies of patients with suspected early Lyme disease, Missouri, 1990–1993. J Infect Dis. 1995;172:470–80.

12A. **Kirkland KB, Klimbo TB, Merriwether RA, et al.** Erythema migrans–like rash illness at a camp in North Carolina: a new tick-borne disease? Arch Intern Med. 1997;157:2635–41.

13. **Steere AC, Taylor E, McHugh GL, Logigian EL.** The overdiagnosis of Lyme disease. JAMA. 1993;269:1812–16.

14. **Dinerman H, Steere AC.** Lyme disease associated with fibromyalgia. Ann Intern Med 1992;117:281–85.

15. **Feinstein AR.** Clinical Epidemiology: The architecture of clinical research. Philadelphia: WB Saunders, 1985.

16. **Aguero-Rosenfeld M, Wormser G, McKenna D, et al.** Human granulocytic ehrlichiosis—a case series from a medical center in New York State, 1995. JAMA. 1995;274:867.

17. **Ley C, Le C, Olshen EM, Reingold AL.** The use of serologic tests for Lyme disease in a prepaid health plan in California. JAMA. 1994;271:460–3.

18. **Eisenberg JM.** Doctors' Decisions and the Cost of Medical Care. The Reasons for Doctors' Practice Patterns and Ways to Change Them. Ann Arbor, MI: Health Administration Press Perspectives, 1986.

19. Morbidity and Mortality Weekly Report 1990;39:397.

20. **Wennberg J, Gittelsohn A.** Small area variations in health care delivery. Science. 1973;182:1102–8.

21. **Wennberg JE, Barnes BA, Zubkoff M.** Professional uncertainty and the problem of supplier-induced demand. Soc Sci Med. 1982;16:811–24.

22. **Keller RB, Soule DN, Wennberg JE, Hanley DF.** Dealing with geographic variations in the use of hospitals. J Bone Joint Surg [Am]. 1990;72:1286–93.

23. **Kassirer JP, Kopelman RI.** Learning Clinical Reasoning. Philadelphia: Williams & Wilkins, 1991.

24. **Davis DA, Thomson MA, Oxman AD, Haynes B.** Evidence for the effectiveness of CME: A review of 50 randomized controlled trials. JAMA. 1992;268:1111–7.

KEY REFERENCES

Eisenberg JM. Doctors' Decisions and the Cost of Medical Care: The Reasons for Doctors' Practice Patterns and Ways to Change Them. Ann Arbor, MI: Health Administration Press Perspectives, 1986.

This book describes various approaches for changing physician practice patterns and discusses what has worked and what has not.

Feder HM, Hunt MS. Pitfalls in the diagnosis and treatment of Lyme disease in children. JAMA. 1995;274:66-8.

Errors in the diagnosis and treatment of Lyme disease in children are common. Frequent pitfalls include misidentifying rashes as erythema migrans, ascribing nonspecific symptoms to Lyme disease, failing to recognize fleeting objective symptoms as Lyme disease, and prescribing inappropriate antibiotic therapy for patients with Lyme disease.

Ley C, Chinh L, Olshen EM, Reingold AL. The use of serologic tests for Lyme disease in a prepaid health plan in California. JAMA. 1994;271:460-3.

In this study, many serologic tests ordered for Lyme disease were performed for reasons other than physician suspicion of Lyme disease in the patient. Patient requests prompted 35% of the serologic tests.

Steere AC, Taylor E, McHugh GL, Logigian EL. The overdiagnosis of Lyme disease. JAMA. 1993;269:1812-6.

This study of a Lyme disease clinic in a university hospital characterizes the most common misdiagnoses of patients referred for suspected Lyme disease. The most common reason for lack of response to antibiotic therapy was misdiagnosis.

Tugwell P, Dennis DI, Weinstein A, et al. Laboratory evaluation in the diagnosis of Lyme disease. Clinical Guideline, Part 2. Ann Intern Med. 1997;127:1109-23.

Clinical

Vignettes

A Man with an Expanding Rash on His Lower Leg, Despite Treatment with Doxycycline

A 62-year-old, insulin-dependent man with diabetes from Denver, Colorado, has a sudden onset of fever and chills and a rash on his left ankle, which he noticed when he awoke. The patient recalls receiving a painful insect bite at this site on the previous day, while camping in the nearby mountains during the Columbus Day weekend.

On physical examination, he is found to be diaphoretic but comfortable and has a temperature of 38 °C, blood pressure of 140/80 mm Hg, and pulse rate of 110 beats/min. A warm, tender, erythematous, "bull's eye" rash, 7 cm in diameter, is noted over the left ankle along with 1+ edema. A left inguinal lymph node is enlarged. An old, well-healed scar is noted on the left leg and on the chest from previous cardiac bypass surgery. The results of the remainder of the physical examination are within the normal range.

Laboratory tests are unremarkable, except for a leukocyte count of 18,000/mm^3 and a glucose level of 280 mg/dL. A tentative diagnosis of Lyme disease is made. Blood samples are drawn to test for *Borrelia burgdorferi* antibodies. The patient is prescribed doxycycline, 100 mg orally twice per day, and told to return if his condition does not improve.

The next day he is admitted to a nearby emergency department with symptoms of an expanding painful and swollen rash, a higher fever, and severe malaise and weakness. The patient is noted to be diaphoretic and appears toxic. His temperature is 39.2 °C; he has a pulse rate of 120 beats/min, and blood pressure of 110/20 mm Hg. The rash on his ankle has now grown to 15 cm and is tender and hot to the touch. Abnormal laboratory test results include a leukocyte count of 32,000/mm^3, glucose level of 400 mg/dL, sodium level of 130 mEq/L, blood urea nitrogen of 30 mg/dL, and creatinine of 1.8 mg/dL.

■ QUESTION

What disease could this expanding rash be caused by?

Bacterial cellulitis is diagnosed, and the patient is admitted and treated with intravenous first-generation cephalosporin. A blood culture obtained on admission grows *Staphylococcus aureus*. His leukocyte count returns to normal, and his fever resolves within 48 hours of treatment. His rash is nearly gone after 1 week of treatment with antibiotics. His initial serologic test for Lyme disease was positive; an immunoblot had several bands reactive with *B. burgdorferi* proteins but did not meet the CDC criteria for a positive blot.

■ **COMMENT**

This patient's illness was initially attributed to Lyme disease, despite the lack of epidemiologic and clinical evidence to support this diagnosis. Lyme disease is not endemic in the Denver area (as opposed to parts of the northeastern, middle Atlantic, and upper midwestern states). Erythema migrans (EM) is also quite rare in October, even in endemic areas, because nymphal-stage deer ticks (which account for the overwhelming majority of cases of Lyme disease) are generally not active after early August. Adult deer ticks (which are active during the autumn and other times of year in endemic areas) are large enough that persons typically remove them before they can transmit infection. Although this patient recalls a painful "insect bite," the bite of a deer tick is usually asymptomatic.

The sudden appearance of a tender rash associated with edema and fever should suggest bacterial cellulitis. The patient's previous saphenous vein surgery and diabetes could each independently put him at risk for this illness. The "bull's eye" rash is *not* specific for EM. Leukocytosis, which is observed in this patient, is common in patients with bacterial cellulitis but rare in Lyme disease.

Despite receiving doxycycline, the patient has further progression of illness. The rapid development of a toxic illness is rare in Lyme disease and should suggest another diagnosis (although some patients with EM who are coinfected with *B. burgdorferi* and other tick-borne pathogens, such as the agent of human granulocytic ehrlichiosis or *Babesia microti*) may be more ill than patients with Lyme disease alone. Although staphylococcal cellulitis may fail to respond to treatment with any *oral* antimicrobial agent, doxycycline should not be prescribed for a patient in whom this entity is likely. Conversely, first-generation cephalosporins, although effective in the treatment of streptococcal and staphylococcal cellulitis, have little activity against *B. burgdorferi* and should not be used in patients with EM. For patients in whom EM cannot easily be distinguished from cellulitis, and in whom treatment with oral agents is appropriate, we typically choose amoxicillin-clavulanate or cefuroxime axetil, which are effective against the etiologic bacteria causing both processes.

The negative immunoblot for *B. burgdorferi* is not surprising, given the low pretest probability for Lyme disease. A Lyme disease assay should not have been ordered, because a positive test result for Lyme disease in such a setting is usually inaccurate. False-positive serologic results for Lyme disease have been associated with syphilis, parvovirus, mononucleosis, rheumatoid arthritis, endocarditis, and other entities. In an area highly endemic for Lyme disease, an EM rash alone is cause for empiric antibiotic therapy; Lyme serologic tests are not necessary for routine cases and should be reserved for a research setting or atypical rashes (in which convalescent serologic testing may be helpful).

■ CONCLUSION

In a person from an area not endemic for Lyme disease, Lyme disease is an unlikely cause of an expanding erythematous rash.

Nadelman RB, Wormser GP. Erythema migrans and early Lyme disease. *Am J Med.* 1995;98(suppl 4A):15S–24S.

Robert B. Nadelman, MD

A Woman with Worsening Symptoms on Initiation of Antibiotics, Followed by Erythema and Paresthesias

A 37-year-old woman from Phoenix, Arizona, develops arthralgias, myalgias, malaise, fatigue, and headache 8 days after returning from a 2-week summer vacation in Westchester County, New York. She denies a history of a tick bite or rash and says that she did not go camping or walking in the woods.

Physical examination reveals that the woman is afebrile and healthy appearing and has a supple neck. There is no evidence of joint abnormalities. A 16 × 16 cm circular lesion with a uniform pink color and a central eschar is noted over the right buttock and lower back. A diagnosis of erythema migrans (EM) is made. Blood samples are drawn to test for antibodies to *B. burgdorferi*, and the patient is prescribed doxycycline, 100 mg orally twice per day for 2 weeks.

During the first day of treatment, the patient's rash intensifies in color, and she experiences worsening headache, myalgia, and fever. She subsequently feels better and the rash resolves within a few days. Serologic testing for Lyme disease is negative. On the last day of antibiotic treatment, the patient returns, complaining of a burning sensation on the back of her hands. She fears she is developing Lyme neuropathy. On physical examination, it is found that the dorsal aspects of both hands and wrists appear erythematous.

■ QUESTION

What is a likely explanation for the course of this patient's illness?

The physician reassures the patient that she has had an adverse reaction to doxycycline, and recommends that she avoid the sun and use over-the-counter analgesics, as needed. The patient's symptoms resolve in a few days. She remains well.

■ COMMENT

This patient developed EM after visiting a region in which Lyme disease occurs commonly, although she resides in a nonendemic area. Most deer tick bites in suburban locales such as Westchester County, New York, are believed to be acquired by persons at their homes rather than through hiking or camping. Activities such as gardening, raking leaves, or attending a lawn barbecue may place persons at risk for acquiring Lyme disease.

The fact that this patient is unaware of any tick bite or rash is not surprising. Unrecognized bites appear to be responsible for more than two thirds of cases of EM. Because significant local symptoms (i.e., pain or pruritus) are generally absent at the sites of the tick bite and EM, a rash may easily be missed if it occurs on a part of the body that is usually covered (e.g., the buttocks or the back). The absence of central clearing is typical of EM cases in the United States. Central clearing is more likely to be present in rashes of long duration.

The patient's physician correctly chose to treat empirically for Lyme disease without awaiting the results of a blood test. More than half of patients with EM are initially seronegative, although more than 80% will ultimately develop antibodies to *B. burgdorferi*. The clinical worsening of the patient's condition on the first day of treatment is consistent with a Jarisch-Herxheimer reaction, which may occur in approximately 15% of patients with EM. Although the mechanism has not been completely elucidated, it is thought to result from the rapid destruction of spirochetes and is also observed in syphilis, relapsing fever, and leptospirosis. Treatment is symptomatic.

The patient received doxycycline for 2 weeks. Although some physicians believe that longer courses of therapy are necessary for patients with EM, there are no convincing data to support this practice. The only published prospective trial addressing the effect of varying durations of oral antimicrobials failed to detect a difference in outcome between 10 and 20 days of treatment with tetracycline. Outcome at 1 year was similar in a separate retrospective study comparing patients who received treatment with doxycycline for 14 days with patients who received it for 20 days. It is our practice to treat patients with EM for 2 weeks.

This patient's symptoms at the end of her therapy are a result of a photosensitivity reaction associated with doxycycline. Patients who cannot avoid sun exposure may be treated with amoxicillin, 500 mg three times per day (if human granulocytic ehrlichiosis is not considered likely). Those receiving doxycycline should be advised to avoid strong sunlight and to protect sun-exposed areas of the body with clothing (e.g., hats and long sleeves and pants) and sunblock.

■ **CONCLUSION**

The timing and distribution of this patient's rash (occurring after antibiotic therapy) suggest a photosensitivity reaction to antibiotics.

Aguero-Rosenfeld ME, Nowakowski J, Bittker S, et al. Evolution of the serologic response to *Borrelia burgdorferi* in treated patients with culture-confirmed erythema migrans. J Clin Microbiol. 1996;34:1–9.

Nadelman RB, Nowakowski J, Forseter G, et al. The clinical spectrum of early Lyme borreliosis in patients with culture-confirmed erythema migrans. Am J Med. 1996;100:502–8.

Wormser GP. Lyme disease: insights into the use of antimicrobials for prevention and treatment in the context of experience with other spirochetal infections. Mt Sinai J Med. 1995;62:188–95.

Robert B. Nadelman, MD

A Man with Leukopenia, Thrombocytopenia, and Mild Liver Abnormalities Occurring After a Recent Tick Bite

A 27-year-old man from Cape Cod, Massachusetts, develops fever, headache, myalgias, malaise, and fatigue over the July 4th weekend. He sees a physician because he is concerned that he might have Lyme disease, since he had a deer tick bite on his calf a week earlier. He denies a history of a rash. Except for a temperature of 38.4 °C, the results of the physical examination, including a skin examination of the entire body, are completely normal. Blood chemistries, a complete blood count, and an assay for antibodies to *B. burgdorferi* are ordered, and the patient is prescribed amoxicillin, 500 mg three times per day, and told to return if his condition does not improve.

He returns after 4 days, without any improvement. His temperature is 38 °C. The results of the remainder of the physical examination are unremarkable. The results of his blood tests are reviewed. Although the hemoglobin is normal, the leukocyte count is 3,400/mm³, and the platelet count is 131,000/mm³. Blood chemistries are normal except for mild elevations of serum aspartate and alanine aminotransferases, and γ-glutamyl transpeptidase. The results of serologic tests for Lyme disease are equivocal.

The patient is told to discontinue the amoxicillin and is prescribed doxycycline, 100 mg twice per day. The patient's symptoms resolve completely over several days. After antibiotic treatment, results of repeat complete blood count and liver function assays are normal. Although an enzyme-linked immunoassay is positive for antibodies to *B. burgdorferi*, an immunoblot does not meet the CDC criteria for positivity and is interpreted as negative. A convalescent serum specimen sent for immunofluorescent antibody assay for the agent of human granulocytic ehrlichiosis is 1:640 (positive).

■ QUESTION

Is this patient's presentation compatible with Lyme disease?

■ COMMENT

This patient develops a febrile systemic illness several days after receiving a recognized "deer tick" bite at a time of year when nymphal-stage deer ticks

(*Ixodes scapularis*) are abundant. Although many persons living in endemic areas are skilled at tick identification, others may mistake scabs, dirt, and other tick species for "deer ticks." Such doubts can be clarified if patients are instructed to bring removed "ticks" to the physician for definitive identification. In any event, more than 95% of *recognized I. scapularis* tick bites do *not* result in transmission of Lyme disease. For this patient from Cape Cod, a tick bite without an EM should serve to emphasize what we already know: that he is at risk for tick-borne diseases, although it is unclear whether *this* particular bite has caused one.

Because no EM is present, several other entities must be considered in addition to Lyme disease in the differential diagnosis, including human granulocytic ehrlichiosis (HGE) and babesiosis (both of which are transmitted by deer ticks), Rocky Mountain spotted fever (transmitted by the dog tick), a viral illness (e.g., enterovirus, parvovirus, mononucleosis, or human immunodeficiency virus), or a noninfectious disease (e.g., vasculitis).

Initially, the patient's physician decides to treat empirically with amoxicillin, presumably for suspected Lyme disease. Although this antibiotic has the advantage of not causing a photosensitivity reaction (important for someone living in a seashore community in July), it has the disadvantage of not providing coverage for HGE.

The patient returns after 4 days without improvement. This fact argues strongly against the diagnosis of Lyme disease. Amoxicillin therapy should be effective in infection with *B. burgdorferi* unless central nervous system infection is present. Most patients with early Lyme disease (who do not have neuroborreliosis) start to note clinical improvement within a few days.

The results of the laboratory tests were also quite unusual for Lyme disease. Leukopenia and thrombocytopenia should suggest another illness (e.g., HGE, babesiosis, Rocky Mountain spotted fever, and viral infections). The results of a peripheral blood smear would be of interest. It is important to look for leukocyte morulae suggestive of HGE infection and intraerythrocytic parasitic forms diagnostic of babesiosis.

Mild liver function abnormalities are observed in this patient. These occur in approximately one third of patients with early Lyme disease and may also be observed in the illnesses mentioned above. It is unclear what to make of an equivocal test result for antibodies to *B. burgdorferi*. Although this is consistent with early Lyme disease or nonspecific reaction, such results should be evaluated further with an immunoblot and repeated several weeks later to determine whether there is an evolution to suggest infection with *B. burgdorferi*.

The lack of clinical response to amoxicillin therapy and the presence of leukopenia, thrombocytopenia, and liver function abnormalities cause the patient's physician to switch the prescribed treatment to doxycycline. This medication could have been started initially, particularly if the results of the complete blood count were available earlier. The patient responds clinically to this treatment. Human granulocytic ehrlichiosis, which may occur separately or together with Lyme disease, is effectively treated with a tetracycline agent such as doxycycline but *not* with β-lactam drugs (e.g., amoxicillin or cefuroxime axetil). Tetracyclines also are effective in the treatment of Rocky Mountain spotted fever and may have some activity against the agent of babesiosis, *Babesia microti.*

A serologic test positive for Lyme disease at first appears to support the diagnosis of Lyme disease. However, the immunoblot suggests that the results of the assay are false-positive. An alternative diagnosis, HGE, is more likely. Recently, evidence has been presented that the agent of HGE itself can cause a false-positive serologic test for Lyme disease (including false-positive immunoblots).

■ CONCLUSION

Atypical clinical features suggest an alternative tick-borne infection—in this case, human granulocytic ehrlichiosis.

Aguero-Rosenfeld ME, Horowitz HW, Wormser GP, et al. Human granulocytic ehrlichiosis (HGE): a case series from a single medical center in New York State. Ann Intern Med. 1996;125:904-8.

Krause PJ, Telford SR III, Spielman A, et al. Concurrent Lyme disease and babesiosis. Evidence for increased severity and duration of illness. JAMA. 1996;275:1657–60.

Wormser GP, Horowitz HW, Nowakowski J, et al. Positive Lyme disease serology in patients with clinical and laboratory evidence of human granulocytic ehrlichiosis. Am J Clin Pathol. 1997;107:142-7.

Robert B. Nadelman, MD

An Elderly Woman with Abrupt Swelling in One Knee

A 73-year-old woman presents in February for evaluation of abrupt onset of swelling in her right knee. She denies any antecedent trauma or previous episode of joint swelling. She has a history of osteoarthritis, principally involving her hands.

The woman lives in northeastern Connecticut and is an avid gardener. She does not spend time in the woods and owns no pets. She denies having a history of a tick bite, skin rash, Bell palsy, or neurologic symptoms. She has noted some stiffness in her joints that has been present for the past several years. Her past medical history is also notable for two previous abdominal surgeries for an ovarian cyst and a hysterectomy, respectively. She is a long-standing 1-pack per day cigarette smoker. She denies alcohol abuse.

On physical examination, she is thin but well appearing. Her weight is 119 lb, blood pressure is 150/90 mm Hg, and pulse rate is 88 beats/min and regular. Her physical examination is notable only for the presence of Heberden and Bouchard nodes in her hands bilaterally, with mild limitation to flexion. Her wrists and shoulders have minimal limitation of motion. She has full range of motion in her elbows, hips, and ankles. She has a large effusion in her right knee that is slightly warm to the touch. A mild flexion deformity is present in her right knee. The left knee is unremarkable. She has mild valgus deformities in her toes but no effusions or soft-tissue swelling.

Review of a radiograph reveals mild medial joint space narrowing and subchondral sclerosis. A large knee effusion is also present.

Laboratory data include a leukocyte count of 5.0×10^9 cells/L, hematocrit of 41.1%, platelet count of 277×10^9 cells/L, with normal electrolytes, liver function studies, and cholesterol level. Uric acid was 6.3 mg/dL. Westergren sedimentation rate is 30 mm/h. Thyroid studies are normal. Serologic testing for Lyme disease revealed an IgM antibody titer of less than 100 and an IgG antibody titer of 1:1600. Western blot analysis notes antibody responses to 25, 31, 39, 41, 60, 66, 75, and 83-kd proteins. Joint fluid analysis reveals erythrocyte count of 4700/mm³, leukocyte of 25,000/mm³ with 75% granulocytes, 15% lymphocytes, and 10% tissue cells. No crystals are noted, and synovial fluid cultures are negative.

■ QUESTION

What is the differential diagnosis?

She receives treatment with oral doxycycline for 30 days. At follow-up, 1 month after completion of antibiotic therapy, she continues to experience stiffness and has evidence of a small right knee effusion. No synovial hypertrophy is palpated. She receives treatment with ibuprofen and is instructed to perform quadriceps-strengthening exercises.

At 6 months' follow-up she has no further recurrences of right knee swelling. Her right knee examination is notable only for the presence of tenderness of the anserine bursa.

■ COMMENT

This elderly woman presents with abrupt swelling in one knee. Although the differential diagnosis of monoarticular arthritis is extensive, three diagnoses in particular need to be considered: degenerative arthritis, crystal-induced arthritis, and Lyme arthritis.

Clearly, this woman has degenerative arthritis in certain joints. On physical examination, she has Heberden and Bouchard nodes, and a radiograph of the swollen right knee showed medial joint-space narrowing and subchondral sclerosis. These are changes typically seen in degenerative arthritis. Although degenerative arthritis may lead to knee swelling, the effusion is typically noninflammatory. Instead, in this patient the joint was warm to the touch, the sedimentation rate was 30 mm/hr, and the joint fluid leukocyte count was 25,000/mm³ with 75% granulocytes. These findings suggest an inflammatory arthritis superimposed on degenerative arthritis of the knee.

In such a patient, it is important to consider the diagnosis of pseudo-gout. This entity, which primarily affects the elderly, is believed to result from the shedding of calcium pyrophosphate crystals into the joint, leading to inflammatory arthritis. Acute attacks most commonly affect the knees, but the wrists or shoulders may also be affected. Thus, the minimal limitation of motion in her wrists and shoulders is consistent with this diagnosis. The *sine qua non* of this entity is the finding of positively birefringent crystals in joint fluid leukocytes, and radiographs of the wrists or knees would be expected to show chondrocalcinosis. However, she had neither finding.

When one joint becomes warm and swollen, even in a patient with known degenerative or inflammatory arthritis, it is important to consider the possibility of infection. The most common bacterial agent to infect joints is *Staphylococcus aureus*. However, this agent typically causes fever, marked pain on joint motion, and a joint fluid leukocyte count in the range of 100,000/mm³, a more severe picture than that described here.

Lyme arthritis, a tick-transmitted spirochetal infection, is usually a less severe form of infectious arthritis that typically causes intermittent attacks of joint swelling and pain in one or a few joints at a time, especially the knee. Joint fluid leukocyte counts are often in the range of 25,000 cells/mm³, and patients are usually not febrile. The diagnosis is based on this characteristic clinical picture, exposure in an endemic area, and serologic confirmation.

This patient lives in northeastern Connecticut, an area highly endemic for Lyme disease. Because the tick that transmits the illness is tiny, most patients do not remember the tick bite, but gardening is an activity that may be associated with this risk. Although the infection usually begins in summer with a characteristic skin lesion (erythema migrans) and flu-like symptoms, this early stage may be asymptomatic, and the illness may present with arthritis months after the initial exposure.

Serologic confirmation should be obtained with a two-test approach of enzyme-linked immunosorbent assay (ELISA) and Western blotting. This patient has an IgG antibody response of 1600 U by ELISA with reactivity with eight spirochetal proteins on Western blot. Although the bands, as listed, include only 3 of the 10 most common IgG bands listed in the CDC criteria (5 are required for a positive response), the blot is probably not read by the laboratory in accordance with the CDC criteria, Thus, this patient's test result should still be interpreted as positive.

Lyme arthritis can usually be treated successfully with a 1-month course of oral doxycycline, which appears to be the case in this patient. Thus, it seems reasonable that this woman had an episode of Lyme arthritis affecting the right knee, superimposed upon low-grade degenerative arthritis of that joint.

■ CONCLUSION

Even in areas endemic for Lyme disease, the differential diagnosis for acute monoarticular arthritis includes degenerative arthritis, crystal-induced arthritis or pseudogout, and septic arthritis, as well as Lyme arthritis.

Kalish RA, Leong JM, Steere AC. Association of treatment resistant chronic Lyme arthritis with HLA-DR4 and antibody reactivity to OspA and OspB of *Borrelia burgdorferi.* Infect Immun. 1993;61:2774–9.

Steere AC, Schoen RT, Taylor E. The clinical evolution of Lyme arthritis. Ann Intern Med. 1987;107:725–31.

Allen C. Steere, MD

A Perimenopausal Woman with Persistent Multijoint Pain and Swelling, Unresponsive to Antibiotics, Following an Untreated Erythema Migrans-like Rash

A 50-year-old woman presents for evaluation of probable Lyme arthritis in December. She states that in May of last year, she noted a red rash on the anterior aspect of her right lower leg. She also noted slight swelling of her right ankle. She states that the swelling improved, but through the course of the summer, she had begun to experience multiple joint pains, particularly after playing tennis and engaging in other strenuous activities. In September of the same year, after bending, her knees "locked." Evaluation performed in October revealed a markedly positive Lyme enzyme-linked immunosorbent assay (ELISA) and Western blot. At that time, she developed some swelling in her left knee and received treatment with doxycycline, 100 mg orally twice per day for 30 days. She also developed a popliteal cyst. She was prescribed a nonsteroidal anti-inflammatory drug after completion of the treatment with doxycycline.

After treatment, she noted profound fatigue, swelling involving her right wrist, and continued swelling of both knees. She continued to take indomethacin, 50 mg three times per day. She denied a history of a tick bite, rash, neurologic symptoms, heart palpitations, or Bell palsy. She did not own any pets and did not spend time in the woods, although she did live in a wooded section of West Hartford, Connecticut.

Her past medical history is significant for a kidney stone 10 years ago. Her medications include estrogen replacement and indomethacin, 50 mg three times per day. She has no known drug allergies. Her family history is significant for osteoarthritis.

On physical examination she is a well-appearing female. Her weight is 155 lb; she has a blood pressure of 122/82 mm Hg, and pulse rate of 64 beats/min and regular. Her skin is clear. The results of the physical examination are normal, with the exception of the musculoskeletal examination. She has swelling in the extensor tendons of her right wrist. The area is noted to be mildly warm to the touch but nonerythematous. She has a small amount of fluid in her right olecranon bursa. In addition, she has bilateral moderately large knee effusions that are associated with increased warmth and synovial thickening. She also has inflammation in the extensor tendons around the right lateral malleolus.

■ QUESTION

What is the differential diagnosis? Is this patient's presentation compatible with Lyme arthritis?

Laboratory testing is notable for a markedly positive Lyme serologic test, with a titer of 1:5120. No protein bands are identified on IgM Western blot analysis. Antibodies to 34, 39, 41, 60, 66, 75, and 83-kd proteins are noted on IgG Western blot. Her sedimentation rate is elevated at 44 mm/h, C reactive protein is 2.5 (0–0.5 mg/dL), HLA-B27 is negative, anti-nuclear antibodies (ANA) is positive with a speckled pattern at a titer of 1:160, extractable nuclear antigens are negative, double-stranded DNA antibodies are negative, rheumatoid factor is negative, and antistreptolysin O titers are negative. Magnetic resonance imaging of her right knee reveals a popliteal cyst.

The patient was retreated with a 2-week course of intravenous ceftriaxone. Four months after completion of therapy, she continued to experience intermittent episodes of joint swelling in her knees.

■ COMMENT

This 50-year-old woman presents for evaluation of probable Lyme arthritis, but various findings suggest that this may not be the correct diagnosis. In contrast with her presentation, the characteristic feature of untreated erythema migrans is gradual expansion of the lesion, and the arthritis does not usually begin until at least weeks later. Moreover, patients with Lyme arthritis usually have complete remission between attacks, whereas she experienced multiple joint pains, particularly after strenuous activity. She then developed swelling of a knee, synovial thickening, and a popliteal cyst, which would be compatible with Lyme arthritis.

On physical examination, she also has swelling of extensor tendons near the wrist and ankle as well as a small amount of fluid in the olecranon bursa. Lyme arthritis may cause tendinitis or bursitis, but attacks are usually intermittent in one location at a time with longer intervening periods of remission.

Moreover, her joint swelling does not respond to treatment with either oral doxycycline or intravenous ceftriaxone therapy. A small percentage of patients with Lyme arthritis, particularly those with HLA-DR4 alleles and antibody reactivity with outer-surface protein A of the spirochete, may have continuous arthritis for months after the antibiotic therapy has presumably eradicated the spirochete from the joint. However, it is unusual for arthritis to develop in new joints after such therapy, which happened in her case.

Her Western blot results do not meet the strict CDC criteria for a positive Western blot, but the test is strongly positive in a range that usually indicates past or present infection with *Borrelia burgdorferi*. Although Lyme disease may not have been the cause of her arthritis, her treatment was such that it should have been sufficient to eradicate the spirochete.

Could the patient have lupus? Although the ANA test is positive in a speckled pattern in a low titer, this is a nonspecific pattern and she lacks other system involvement that would point toward this diagnosis. Seronegative forms of chronic inflammatory arthritis include ankylosing spondylitis, Reiter syndrome, psoriatic arthritis, or arthritis associated with inflammatory bowel disease, but this patient lacks specific findings that would point to these diagnoses. Seronegative rheumatoid arthritis may affect tendons near the wrist and ankles, but the intermittent character of the arthritis and the absence of symmetrical polyarthritis would seem to make this possibility less likely.

Might this patient have a crystal-induced form of chronic inflammatory arthritis? In gouty arthritis, which is caused by monosodium urate crystals, initial attacks are usually monoarticular with few constitutional symptoms. An ankle would be a possible first location, and the surrounding skin may resemble a bacterial cellulitis. Tendons and the olecranon bursa may also be affected. Uric acid kidney stones may be the presenting feature of the disease, particularly in patients with hypercalciuria. In women, gout is unusual before menopause, but it becomes as common as in men after menopause. Another possibility is pseudogout, which is caused by calcium pyrophosphate crystals, but the involvement of tendons, bursa, and skin is more typical of gout.

In this patient, serum and 24-hour urine samples should be analyzed for uric acid and calcium levels. Radiographs of the wrists and knees should be done to determine whether there is chondrocalcinosis. However, the critical test would be a joint fluid analysis with crystal search. If gout or pseudogout is the correct diagnosis, acute attacks should be treated with indomethacin or other nonsteroidal anti-inflammatory agents.

■ CONCLUSION

Multijoint swelling accompanied by tendinitis and bursitis would be an unusual presentation of Lyme arthritis. Alternative diagnoses should be pursued, including systemic lupus erythematosus, seronegative arthropathies, and crystal-induced arthritis (gout or pseudogout).

Steere AC, Schoen RT, Taylor E. The clinical evolution of Lyme arthritis. Ann Intern Med. 1987;107:725–31.

Allen C. Steere, MD

A Previously Healthy 10-year-old Girl with Acute Onset of Complete Heart Block

In July, a previously healthy 10-year-old girl presents to the emergency department with chief symptoms of fatigue on exertion and dizziness for approximately 2 days. She has no history of heart problems, rash, or a tick bite. Her mother notes that she has "felt warm" for the past week.

On physical examination she is pale with a temperature of 37.6 °C. Her blood pressure is 98/64 mm Hg, and her pulse rate is 50 beats/min. She has no rashes and her throat is clear. Her lungs are clear to auscultation and percussion. Her heart examination is notable for bradycardic regular rhythm, and she has a grade II/VI systolic ejection murmur. The results of the abdominal examination are benign. The results of the musculoskeletal and neurologic examinations are normal.

An electrocardiogram showed complete heart block with an escape rhythm of 50 beats/min. The QRS configuration had a predominantly left bundle branch block pattern indicating a ventricular escape rhythm. The atrial rate was approximately 120 beats/min. Echocardiography revealed a morphologically normal heart with excellent contractility. There was slight mitral regurgitation.

Laboratory findings included an leukocyte count of 9800/mm^3 with 6% bands, 63% neutrophils, 26% lymphocytes, 3% monocytes, and 2% eosinophils. Her sedimentation rate was elevated to 60 mm/h. Serologic testing and stool examinations are negative for viral diseases. The results of complement, antinuclear antibody, and streptococcal antibody tests are normal. Serologic tests for Lyme disease are positive for IgM (1:1600) and IgG (1:800).

■ QUESTION

How should this case be managed at this point?

The patient is admitted, placed on cardiac monitoring, and begins receiving intravenous ceftriaxone (2 g/d). After admission her heart rate decreases to approximately 30 beats/min for short periods and she complains of dizziness. Placement of a temporary cardiac pacemaker is considered. She is given a continuous infusion of orciprenaline and her heart rate increased to 60 beats/min. After 4 days, the complete heart block changed to a 2:1 second-degree atrioventricular block. One week after admission she had mainly first-degree atrioventricular block with a PR interval of 0.40 sec. Her heart rate reverted to normal sinus rhythm with a normal PR interval after 2 weeks.

■ COMMENT

The patient is a previously healthy 10-year-old girl with acute onset complete heart block. Heart block in this setting suggests an infectious cause. In such cases, careful epidemiologic inquiry should be made regarding recent trips to or residence in endemic areas for Lyme disease. The presence of associated symptoms of early disseminated Lyme disease, such as a history of a tick bite, expanding skin rash, febrile systemic illness, and seventh nerve palsy, is strong supportive evidence. Alternative causes of heart block, such as acute rheumatic fever, viruses, and other bacterial infections, should be considered.

Acute rheumatic fever (ARF) primarily involves children between the ages of 5 and 15 years. Jones' major criteria include carditis, arthritis, chorea, erythema marginatum, and subcutaneous nodules. Carditis in ARF usually presents as a significant heart murmur, and mitral value involvement is common. In contrast, valvular involvement in Lyme carditis is unusual. Prolongation of the PR interval may be present in both diseases, but complete heart block rarely occurs in ARF, especially without associated valvular involvement and congestive heart failure.

Throat culture and a rapid streptoccoal antigen detection test should be done, especially in children presenting with carditis. In some reported cases of Lyme carditis, elevated antistreptolysin O titers were present and resulted in diagnostic problems. The presence of supportive epidemiologic, clinical, and serologic data may favor one diagnosis over another. Bacterial and viral infectious causes may be ruled out with serologic testing, in the appropriate setting.

Lyme carditis occurs during the acute disseminated phase and typically occurs 3 to 6 weeks after initial infection. As in this case, patients may lack other features of Lyme disease or develop nonspecific symptoms and not seek medical attention before the onset of cardiac symptoms. In general, symptoms suggestive of cardiac involvement occur with high-degree atrioventricular block. It is likely that many cases of first-degree heart block go undetected.

Patients with high-degree heart block should be hospitalized with cardiac monitoring because the degree of heart block may flucuate rapidly and progress from first- to third-degree heart block in a matter of minutes. It is unclear if antibiotics hasten the resolution of heart block; however, in a hospitalized patient, treatment with intravenous antibiotics is indicated to clear the organism and prevent potential serious late sequelae. Ceftriaxone (2 g per day for 14 to 30 days) or penicillin G (20 million U per day for 14 to 30 days) is the antibiotic of choice. Optimum duration of treatment is unknown, and associated clinical manifestations (i.e., neurologic disease) would influence the management decision. A 30-day course of oral therapy with either amoxicillin (500 mg orally three times per day) or doxycycline

(100 mg orally two times per day) may be given to patients with milder disease (PR intervals <0.3 sec).

Additional cardiac intervention such as insertion of a temporary pacemaker is necessary in patients with severe/symptomatic heart block. In younger patients who are not at risk for underlying cardiac disease, agents such as isoprenaline and atropine may be used. Permanent pacemakers are rarely indicated.

It is uncertain if the addition of aspirin or prednisone to antibiotic therapy is of value. Theoretically, prednisone may interfere with the immune system's ability to clear the organism and therefore is not recommended in most cases of carditis. However, some patients have dense heart block that persists for longer than 2 to 4 days despite adequate antibiotic treatment, and in such cases, the addition of steroids or aspirin may decrease the chance of permanent sequelae by reducing the inflammatory response and prevent possible irreversible injury to the cardiac conduction system. A short course of high-dose steroids (prednisone, 1 mg/kg per day) with a quick taper over 1 week can be used.

Recovery from Lyme carditis is complete in almost all cases, regardless of therapy. There have been no reports of progressive heart disease occurring after successful treatment for Lyme carditis. Occasionally, especially in severe cases, recovery may be incomplete. This does not indicate that *Borrelia burgdorferi* is still present in cardiac tissue; rather, permanent injury was sustained despite successful eradication of the organism. There have been case reports of patients requiring permanent pacemakers, but fortunately, it is a rare event. Because of the excellent prognosis, in most cases long-term follow-up with cardiac studies is not necessary.

■ **CONCLUSION**

Patients with Lyme carditis can present quite dramatically. They usually require hospitalization and careful cardiac monitoring for potential serious complications.

McAlister HF, Klementowicz PT, Andrews C, et al. Lyme carditis: an important cause of reversible heart block. Ann Intern Med. 1989:110:339–45.

Steere AC, Batsford WP, Weinberg M, et al. Lyme carditis: cardiac abnormalities of Lyme disease. Ann Intern Med. 1980:93:8–16.

van der Linde MR, Crigns JGM, de Koning J, et al. Range of atrioventricular conduction disturbances in Lyme borreliosis: a report of four cases and review of other published reports. Br Heart J. 1990:63:162–8.

Janine Evans, MD

Lyme Disease as a Possible Cause of Attention-Deficit Disorder and Persistent Knee Pain in an 11-year-old Boy

An 11-year old boy has a 2-year history of intermittent knee pain as well as a long history of inattention, distractibility, and daydreaming. In July 1995, he was diagnosed as having attention-deficit disorder. Osgood–Schlatter disease and chondromalacia of the patella were diagnosed in October 1995. He was treated with exercises and nonsteroidal anti-inflammatory drugs. After attending a seminar on attention-deficit disorders, his mother wondered if Lyme disease could be the cause of her son's condition.

His symptoms included headaches, recurrent sore throat, nausea, and dizziness. He experienced a great deal of pain in his knees, especially with exercise. He had no history of a tick bite, erythema migrans, facial nerve palsy, joint swelling, paresthesias, motor weakness, or heart palpitations. He lives in a wooded area in which Lyme disease is highly endemic.

A serologic test for Lyme disease was done at the mother's request and returned negative; however, a repeat test done at a different laboratory was positive.

The patient received treatment with amoxicillin for 3 weeks beginning in May 1996, followed by a second course of treatment with amoxicillin in June 1996. After his second course of treatment, he felt somewhat better. The only persistent symptom was sore knees. His attention-deficit disorder was unchanged.

The patient presents for further evaluation of possible Lyme disease. On physical examination, he is well-appearing and in no acute distress. The results of his HEENT examination are unremarkable. His neck is supple without lymphadenopathy. His lungs are clear, and his heart has a regular rate and rhythm with no murmurs. His abdomen is soft and nontender with normal bowel sounds. There is no evidence of either peripheral cyanosis or edema. His musculoskeletal examination is significant for very mild soft tissue swelling and tenderness over both tibial tuberosities. The results of the neurologic examination are normal.

Laboratory studies included a leukocyte count of 5900/mm^3 with a normal differential. His hemoglobin is 13.9 g/dL, and his hematocrit is 39.3%. Monospot test, rheumatoid factor, anti-streptolysin O titer, and antinuclear antibody tests are negative. The erythrocyte sedimentation rate is 3 mm/h. Initial Lyme serologies are interpreted as being borderline positive but were negative when they were repeated.

■ QUESTION

Is Lyme disease a likely cause of this child's cognitive and joint complaints?

■ COMMENT

This child's initial symptoms were very nonspecific and could have been caused by several different conditions. It is important to note that all of the symptoms were subjective. There were no objective abnormalities that are typically associated with Lyme disease. The pain in the knees was associated with activity, and there were no objective signs of inflammation (e.g., swelling of a joint, which might indicate synovitis). In addition to organic causes of his symptoms, psychological stress and anxiety must be considered. As in adults, children often manifest anxiety through physical symptoms.

Regarding the serologic tests for Lyme disease, in the absence of either specific symptoms or objective signs of Lyme disease, the probability that this child has Lyme disease is extremely low (<1%). The specificity of even the best serologic tests for Lyme disease is far from 100% (and many of the prepackaged commercial kits that are widely used to test for antibodies have poor specificity). The accuracy of serologic tests can be improved by the use of a two-step procedure in which a positive test by enzyme-linked immunosorbent assay is confirmed with a Western immunoblot.

Nevertheless, the positive predictive value of a positive serologic test (even of relatively accurate tests performed at reference laboratories) is poor if the "pretest probability" (the probability of Lyme disease before the result of the test is known) is low. In this setting (i.e., a patient with a pretest probability of Lyme disease of <1%), >95% of positive serologic tests will yield false-positive results. Several investigators have documented the high proportion of patients seen at referral centers who are misdiagnosed as having Lyme disease, and this can be attributed, at least in part, to the indiscriminant use of serologic tests.

After receiving a second course of treatment, the patient reported that he "felt better." It is common for nonspecific symptoms of persons without Lyme disease to "improve" after they receive treatment with antibiotics. First, the "placebo effect" is a well-recognized phenomenon. In addition, over time, nonspecific symptoms of whatever cause often improve, at least temporarily (though subsequent "relapse" also is common).

On the current examination, again, the only objective abnormalities are the swelling and tenderness over the tibial tuberosities, which are consistent with Osgood–Schlatter disease. The serologic test for Lyme disease ultimately is negative.

Because the nonspecific symptoms that this child has have been chronic, if they are caused by Lyme disease, the Lyme disease presumably would be late stage. Antibodies to *Borrelia burgdorferi* are virtually always positive in this stage of the disease. Consequently, if the tests for antibody truly are negative (false-negative tests are much less common than false-positive tests), it virtually rules out Lyme disease as a cause of the symptoms. This is not true for early-stage Lyme disease, in which the signs and symptoms may precede seroconversion. Early treatment with antibiotics in patients with early Lyme disease may ablate the antibody response so that such patients may never develop antibodies. However, once antibodies do develop (as they would in late Lyme disease), the antibodies persist despite antibiotic treatment.

■ **CONCLUSION**

In patients presenting with nonspecific symptoms, the positive predictive value of serologic testing for Lyme disease is low.

Seltzer EG, Shapiro ED. Misdiagnosis of Lyme disease: when not to order serologic tests. Pediatr Infect Dis J. 1996;15:762–3.

Sigal LH, Patella SJ. Lyme arthritis as the incorrect diagnosis in pediatric and adolescent fibromyalgia. Pediatrics. 1992;90:523–8.

Steere AC, Taylor E, McHugh GL, et al. The overdiagnosis of Lyme disease. JAMA. 1993;269:1812–26.

Eugene D. Shapiro, MD

A 7-year-old Boy with Facial Palsy Beginning 9 Months after Receiving a Tick Bite

A 7-year-old boy from Vermont presents for evaluation of facial palsy and possible Lyme disease. During the previous summer, he experienced a flu-like illness associated with a bumpy rash in his axilla. At the time, he had been vacationing with his family in Cape Cod. In retrospect, the parents recall removing a small tick from his leg during that vacation. His symptoms resolved completely over a 5- to 7-day period.

He was well until March, when he developed a droop of the right side of the face. He had had an infection of the upper respiratory tract that began the week before, although he had not had fever or other systemic symptoms.

The results of a urinary antigen test for Lyme disease are positive. Treatment with azithromycin is started before the child is referred for further evaluation.

■ QUESTION

Do the clinical manifestations and laboratory data support a diagnosis of Lyme facial palsy in this child?

The results of this patient's physical examination are normal except for a mild, peripheral palsy of the right facial nerve that apparently was beginning to resolve. An antibody test for Lyme disease, sent to a reference laboratory, is returned negative. Treatment with azithromycin is discontinued, and the facial nerve palsy resolves completely.

■ COMMENT

It is unlikely that the original illness in this child was Lyme disease. Erythema migrans is a flat rash (vesicles may develop in the center of the rash, but that is uncommon). The rash in this child is not described as annular (which is characteristic of EM) and, if untreated, EM usually lasts for several weeks. The history of a tick bite serves only to indicate that the child was exposed to ticks but not necessarily infected with *Borrelia burgdorferi*.

Even if the initial illness was Lyme disease, it is unlikely that the current facial palsy is related. Facial palsy is a manifestation of early disseminated Lyme disease, which usually develops 3 to 8 weeks after the initial infection. If this child were to develop manifestations that resulted from untreated Lyme disease the year before, one would expect that the child would develop arthritis, not facial nerve palsy. Although recent infection with *B. burgdorferi* certainly is possible, the epidemiologic history argues against this. First, the child lives in Vermont, where Lyme disease is rare, and second, the tick bite would have occurred in either January or February, which is unlikely in most areas of the northeastern United States, especially in Vermont.

No reliable tests are available for antigens of *B. burgdorferi* in the urine. Tests that have been marketed have a very high rate of false-positive results, and some have been removed from the market by the manufacturer.

The medication of choice treating Lyme disease in a child of this age is amoxicillin. There are only limited data on the use of azithromycin to treat Lyme disease in adults, and there are no published clinical trials of its use in children. Those data suggest that azithromycin is no better, and may be worse, than the conventional oral agents, amoxicillin and doxycycline. Because antimicrobial agents do not affect the outcome of facial nerve palsy caused by Lyme disease (it usually resolves completely regardless of whether antimicrobial treatment is given), the primary goal of treatment is to prevent late Lyme disease (Lyme arthritis). There are no published data on the efficacy of azithromycin in preventing late-stage Lyme disease—another reason to avoid using this drug in a child with Lyme disease.

■ CONCLUSION

The atypical original illness, the late occurrence of neurologic involvement, and the unreliability of the laboratory test results do not support a diagnosis of Lyme disease.

Gerber MA, Shapiro ED, Burke GS, et al. Lyme disease in children in southeastern Connecticut. N Engl J Med. 1996;335:1270–4.

Luft BJ, Dattwyler RJ, Johnson RC, et al. Azithromycin compared with amoxicillin in the treatment of erythema migrans: a double-blind, randomized, controlled trial. Ann Intern Med. 1996;124:785–91.

Eugene D. Shapiro, MD

Chronic Recurring Symptoms Despite Antibiotic Therapy

A 46-year-old man presents for evaluation of possible Lyme disease. The patient reported that he was generally well until the previous summer. In early July, he had a flu-like illness with myalgias, head congestion, malaise, some neck stiffness, and a rash over the right elbow. The rash spread to approximately 5 cm in diameter. At that time, he was seen by his internist and was diagnosed as having possible Lyme disease. He received treatment with doxycycline, 100 mg twice per day for 2 weeks. His symptoms persisted, and he continued the treatment for a total of 28 days.

By the time he completed the therapy, he felt better but still had some fatigue and malaise. Within weeks, however, his other symptoms returned. He was prescribed a second course of doxycycline for 2 weeks later in the summer. The symptoms again recurred after the second course of therapy was completed. He was treated again in September with azithromycin, 250 mg for 2 weeks.

In December his symptoms recurred and he was concerned that he might have Lyme disease. He received an additional course of azithromycin. He reported that his symptoms consisted of "congestion of the left nostril, tingling of the fingertips and lips, and a sense that his feet were numb." He also experienced muscle cramps and found that he had "no energy" if he exercised.

Lyme serologic tests performed at the initial visit in July were negative. A repeat study in September was interpreted as positive; Lyme (IgG and IgM) enzyme-linked immunosorbent assay was 1.34 (<0.80 is negative). Repeat IgM and IgG serologic tests performed in December were equivocal.

His past medical history is unremarkable, although he reports that a friend had been "crippled" by Lyme disease.

On the current examination, his skin is clear. The head, ears, eyes, nose, and throat are normal. The neck is supple, and there is no lymphadenopathy. The lungs are clear and the cardiac examination reveals an S_1 and S_2. The abdomen is soft. There is no hepatosplenomegaly. The results of the musculoskeletal examination are normal, and the neurologic examination was without focal findings. The results of a Lyme serologic test performed at the time of evaluation were negative.

■ QUESTION

Is a course of intravenous antibiotics warranted?

■ COMMENT

The head congestion associated with the patient's initial illness in July makes the diagnosis less likely to be Lyme disease; coryza and sinus congestion are quite uncommon in Lyme disease. If this were Lyme disease, his receiving a full 28-day course of doxycycline was, in terms of drug, dose, and duration, ample to kill *Borrelia burgdorferi*. The fact that within a few days after treatment was discontinued he had recrudescence of his symptoms cannot be viewed as evidence that the infection was active. *B. burgdorferi* is a very slow-growing organism, so that the quick return of symptoms is unlikely to indicate regrowth of a small number of residual organisms to a significant biomass. Further antibiotic treatment also was of no avail.

Of note, at no time were there any objective findings of Lyme disease or of any inflammatory disease. Lyme disease is associated with objective evidence of tissue damage—in the skin, heart, nerves, or brain. If there is no objective evidence of tissue damage, the diagnosis of Lyme disease should be called into question.

The original diagnosis is suggested by the finding of a rash on the right elbow. Erythema migrans is usually found at the midriff, groin, knee, and axilla. Erythema migrans over the elbow is unusual, although not impossible. It would have been useful to know how long the rash lasted. If it persisted until the doctor's visit, did it resolve during antibiotic therapy? Finally, we do not know if this patient lived in or had recently visited an endemic area.

Symptoms recurred after treatment, but they are not of a pattern that suggests Lyme disease. Numbness and tingling can be seen in Lyme disease, but the bilaterally symmetrical distribution should suggest other causes (e.g., diabetic neuropathy). Lack of energy is ubiquitous in our society; isolated fatigue in the absence of objective findings should not suggest Lyme disease, acute or "chronic."

If, in fact, the patient had Lyme disease in July, the negative test at the initial visit would be of no value, as results of testing done within the first few days of the infection are often negative. The test that was done in September, without confirmation by Western blot analysis, cannot be interpreted. If this is a false-positive enzyme-linked immunosorbent assay (ELISA) (positive ELISA, negative blot), the result is of no consequence. If this is a true-positive (positive ELISA, positive blot), it is a marker of previous exposure and nothing more. Persisting seropositivity is not evidence of active or ongoing infection; it merely represents previous exposure.

The fact that a friend was "crippled" by Lyme disease lends a psychological overlay to the case, suggesting that the patient may ascribe great importance to his symptoms and to his belief that they are caused by Lyme disease. Such patients may become hypervigilant. The very symptoms of anxiety and stress may, by this process, be interpreted as indicating real disease.

The results of the current physical examination are unremarkable, compatible with the possibility that this patient is interpreting symptoms and thereby magnifying them. The negative serologic test at the time of this evaluation cannot be interpreted as evidence for or against previous infection.

There is no reason that this patient should receive treatment with further antibiotics. He should be reassured that he does not have and probably never has had Lyme disease. Some patients are very unwilling to be disabused of a diagnosis of Lyme disease. Many such patients do not even want to consider that their symptoms may be caused by stress, anxiety, or an alternative diagnosis such as fibromyalgia, a common mimic of "chronic" Lyme disease.

■ CONCLUSION

When there are no objective clinical findings indicating active infection from Lyme disease, repeated courses of antibiotic treatment are unwarranted unless required for an alternative diagnosis.

Sigal LH. Persisting complaints attributed to Lyme disease: possible mechanisms and implications for management. Am J Med. 1994;96:365–74.

Sigal LH. Special Article: diagnostic and management pitfalls in Lyme disease. Arthritis Rheum. 1997 (In press.)

Leonard H. Sigal, MD

A 16-year-old Girl with Long-standing, Widespread Joint Pain, Headaches, Nausea, and Excessive Tiredness

A 16-year-old girl had been experiencing profound fatigue, migratory daily headaches lasting for hours, dizziness, nausea, and joint pain since the age of 12 years. Her joint pain involved her knees, ankles, wrists, temporomandibular joints, back, and sometimes hands. In addition, she complained about the first carpometacarpal joint of her thumb and occasionally the metacarpophalangeal joints. There was minimal swelling, if any, but a significant degree of pain.

She noted a rash on the anterior part of her neck at the beginning of her symptoms but did not give a clear description of erythema migrans. She did not distinctly remember a tick bite. She also did not experience facial palsy, carditis, or frank swelling in her joints. She does live in a wooded area inhabited by numerous deer. An initial Lyme serologic test was negative, but repeat serologic studies performed at a different laboratory were reported to be positive.

After evaluation of these symptoms, she was diagnosed as having Lyme disease and treated for 4 to 5 months with oral antibiotics, beginning with doxycycline and followed by amoxicillin and cefixime. She had minimal benefit from the antibiotic treatment and therefore was prescribed intravenous ceftriaxone for 1 month. Her intravenous therapy was complicated by the development of pseudomembranous colitis, which was treated with metronidazole. After antibiotic therapy was completed, she had only minimal improvement.

Three years later she received treatment with azithromycin. She was unable to continue treatment owing to gastrointestinal upset. She then received amoxicillin for 2 weeks, but she developed hives and the treatment was therefore discontinued. She stated that while on and off antibiotics, she never felt completely better.

Her past medical history is one of normal growth and development until the age of 12 years, when her symptoms began. Her menses began at age 11 years and were complicated by significant dysmenorrhea. She had been taking birth control pills to control her symptoms. She also stated that she would sleep 3 to 5 hours every day after school and then went to bed at 10 p.m., arising at 7 a.m. each morning feeling very tired.

On physical examination, she is thin but well appearing and in no acute distress. Her weight is 98 lb, blood pressure 106/76 mm Hg, and pulse rate 76 beats/min and regular. Her skin is clear. She does have a small, tender, superficial subcutaneous nodule under her left axilla that has a cystic component. The results of the rest of her skin examination are normal. Her abdomen is soft and nontender with normal active bowel sounds. She does not have an enlarged liver or palpable spleen.

Examination of her extremities reveals evidence of a livedo pattern on the dorsum of her hands and feet bilaterally that disappeared with warming. Her musculoskeletal examination shows no evidence of synovitis in any of her joints. She does have mild tenderness with compression of her patellofemoral joint. Her neurologic examination is significant for 5/5 strength throughout, 2+ reflexes in both her upper and lower extremities. Her toes are down-going. She has normal vibratory sense and a normal tandem gait, negative Romberg sign, and normal cerebellar signs. Her cranial nerves are intact and symmetric.

■ QUESTION

What is the differential diagnosis?

Review of her laboratory data reveals normal thyroid function studies, a normal complete blood count, and a sedimentation rate of 10 mm/h. As noted above, the Lyme serologic tests show a recent Lyme serologic test that is negative and a Western blot reveals a 41-kd protein band. Hepatitis screen, rapid plasma reagin (RPR), lupus anticoagulant, anticardiolipin antibodies, antinuclear antibodies (ANA), cold agglutinins, cryoglobulins, cytomegalovirus (CMV) titers, and Epstein-Barr titers are negative. Prothrombin time (PT) and partial thromboplastin time (PTT) are normal. Radiographs of her chest and wrists are normal. Computed tomography of her head is normal. The results of ophthalmologic and ENT examinations are also normal.

■ COMMENT

This patient presents with a 4-year history of nonspecific symptoms. Arthralgia is described, although little or no evidence of true inflammatory joint disease is found. Overall, the clinical findings do not explicitly suggest Lyme disease; the rash did not suggest erythema migrans, and she had no other objective findings to suggest infection with *Borrelia burgdorferi*. Despite a negative serologic test, the diagnosis of Lyme disease was made. In a patient who has had symptoms for 4 years, despite more than adequate antibiotic therapy, one must maintain a certain skepticism about the initial diagnosis of Lyme disease; in our experience, the most common cause for lack of response to adequate therapy is initial misdiagnosis. Note also that this young woman also has had many serious side effects of antibiotic therapy.

Despite courses of proper antibiotics, the patient remains symptomatic, describing symptoms (except for her arthralgias) that are not classic for or suggestive of later manifestations of Lyme disease. Her fatigue is notable. Her excessive sleeping suggests an underlying sleep disorder. Noninflammatory musculoskeletal pain in combination with a sleep disorder suggests the possibility of fibromyalgia, a syndrome commonly mistaken for "chronic" Lyme disease.

The current physical examination reveals no objective physical findings. For her physical examination to be totally normal suggests that infection with *B. burgdorferi* may not be present.

The sedimentation rate (ESR) in Lyme disease is usually not very accelerated; the value of the normal ESR here is to reassure the evaluating physician that there is a low probability of an occult inflammatory disease. Serologic testing for anti–*B. burgdorferi* antibodies is negative. However, after all the antibiotics this patient has received, the negative serologic test is of no real consequence. Certainly the finding of livedo reticularis suggests the possibility of the anticardiolipin antibody syndrome, even in the absence of any prior clinical features of this syndrome. Some of these patients have lupus or a lupus-like syndrome; no evidence of this is present in the current case, either. Thus, results of the anticardiolipin antibody test, lupus anticoagulant, PT, PTT, RPR, and ANA were all reasonable and reassuring. Livedo reticularis can be caused by cryoglobulinemia and vasculitis affecting medium-sized muscular arteries. The negative serologic tests for hepatitis B and C indicate that in this patient there is no viral cause for polyarteritis nodosa. Her ongoing distal joint pains could be considered compatible with sarcoidosis (bilateral ankle pain) or pulmonary hypertrophic osteoarthropathy (pain caused by possible distal tibia/fibula and radius/ulna periostitis) so that chest and wrist radiographs are also reasonable. The finding of IgM anti-CMV or anti-Epstein–Barr antibodies would be evidence of recent infection with one of these viruses; however, such a finding would not explain a 4-year history of this patient's symptoms.

Thus, physical examination and laboratory evaluation fail to provide a basis for a diagnosis of Lyme disease, a diagnosis that was only vaguely suggested by the patient's history and that was made less likely by her subsequent course. Further evaluation, with a focus on sleep disorder and possible fibromyalgia, is in order.

■ CONCLUSION

In patients who present with arthralgias after receiving antibiotic therapy, alternative diagnoses, such as a sleep disorder with possible fibromyalgia, autoimmune disease, or viral illnesses, should be considered. Appropriate laboratory tests may be useful in making the diagnosis.

Sigal LH. Summary of the first one hundred patients seen at a Lyme disease referral center. Am J Med. 1990;88:577–81.

Sigal LH. Persisting complaints attributed to chronic Lyme disease: possible mechanisms and implications for management. Am J Med. 1994;96:365–74.

Sigal LH, Patella SJ. Lyme arthritis as the incorrect diagnosis in pediatric and adolescent fibromyalgia. Pediatrics. 1992;90:523–8.

Leonard H. Sigal, MD

A Pregnant Woman with Possible Tick Bite

A 32-year-old woman who is 8 months pregnant presents for treatment of Lyme disease. She lives in an area endemic for Lyme disease and had removed a deer tick 1 day before presentation. She is uncertain how long the tick had been attached. She denies having fever, skin rash, or other constitutional symptoms. She is allergic to penicillin.

Her physical examination is notable for a palpable uterine fundus associated with a pregnancy of approximately 36 weeks. The rest of her examination is normal.

■ QUESTION

Is prophylactic therapy advisable? If so, which antibiotic would be appropriate?

■ COMMENT

This woman has a strong possibility of exposure to Lyme disease, although the likelihood of getting Lyme disease from a known tick bite, when the tick is removed and engorged, is only 8% according to the only large-scale study of tick bite risk. Nevertheless, there is some risk.

There is no evidence of Lyme disease at this time, but erythema migrans can be delayed by as many as 30 days after tick bite. Thus, the question is: "to treat or not to treat."

If one were to be concerned about fetal anomalies caused by Lyme disease, the organs of this woman's baby have been formed and growing for months. Premature labor has been reported in pregnancies complicated by Lyme disease, but the real risk of this happening and the risk if it were to occur are probably small.

Many clinicians would treat her, if only to allow her peace of mind. The choice of antibiotic is somewhat complicated by the history of penicillin allergy. Many patients report having a penicillin allergy but describe manifestations of stomach upset, nausea, diarrhea, vaginitis, or oral thrush that are not allergy but instead adverse effects from antibiotic treatment. A 1-month course of erythromycin or cefuroxime axetil could be tried. The newer macrolide antibiotics (e.g., azithromycin and clarithromycin) are of unproven value in the treatment of Lyme disease and are certainly more expensive than erythromycin. Because they offer no advantage, they should not be used routinely.

■ CONCLUSION

The need for antibiotic prophylaxis in late pregnancy is questionable, but erythromycin or cefuroxime axetil could be used safely.

Dennis DT, Meltzer MI. Antibiotic prophylaxis after tick bite. Lancet. 1997;350: 1191–2.

Strobino BA, Williams CL, Abid S, et al. Lyme disease and pregnancy outcome: a prospective study of 2,000 prenatal patients. Am J Obstet Gynecol. 1993;169:367–74.

Williams CL, Strobino B, Weinstein A, et al. Maternal Lyme disease and congenital malformations: a cord blood serosurvey in endemic and control areas. Paediatr Perinat Epidemiol. 1995;9:320–30.

Leonard H. Sigal, MD

A Pregnant Woman with Possible Erythema Migrans

A 26-year-old woman who is approximately 13 weeks pregnant presents for evaluation of an expanding erythematous skin lesion on her anterior thigh. She had been hiking in the woods 1 week before developing the skin rash. She had not noted a tick bite. On the day before presentation, she developed a fever of 38.3 °C, nausea, mild headache, and profound fatigue. She denies facial drooping, stiff neck, or heart palpitations.

On physical examination she is well appearing. Her temperature is 100.5 °F, pulse rate 90 beats/min, blood pressure 110/70 mm Hg, and respiration 18 breaths/min. Her examination is normal with the exception of a circular, erythematous, macular lesion on her anterior left thigh measuring approximately 5 × 4 cm.

■ **QUESTION**

What is the appropriate antibiotic regimen?

■ **COMMENT**

Based on the description of the rash, erythema migrans is a high likelihood, unless this woman was hiking in a nonendemic area. Because the rash is asymptomatic, it is unlikely to have been the result of a spider bite. She has developed fever, headache, and fatigue but has no objective findings to suggest early disseminated disease. Thus, based on the history, early localized Lyme disease is very likely.

The next step is to prescribe treatment. Oral antibiotics are in order, because there is no evidence of dissemination and there is no proof that intravenous therapy improves the outcome for either mother or fetus. A 1-month course of amoxicillin is recommended. Alternatively, erythromycin or cefuroxime axetil could be tried. The newer macrolide antibiotics, azithromycin and clarithromycin, are of unproven value in the treatment of Lyme disease and are more expensive than erythromycin. Because they offer no advantage, they should not be used routinely.

The outcome of pregnancy complicated by Lyme disease is a major concern here. The current thinking is that adequate treatment will avoid an adverse outcome. A number of good prospective epidemiologic studies have found no evidence that Lyme disease has an adverse effect on the fetus, although none absolutely rules out the possibility that the infection may adversely affect the fetus. The ramifications of this infection are not proven, but if there is an effect on the fetus it must be relatively infrequent.

■ CONCLUSION

Oral antibiotics are appropriate in early localized Lyme disease, even in pregnancy. Intravenous antibiotics should be considered in cases of disseminated disease.

Gerber MA, Zalneraitis EL. Childhood neurologic disorders and Lyme disease during pregnancy. Pediatr Neurol. 1994;11:41–3.

Strobino BA, Williams CL, Abid S, ct al. Lyme disease and pregnancy outcome: a prospective study of 2,000 prenatal patients. Am J Obstet Gynecol. 1993;169:367–74.

Williams CL, Strobino B, Weinstein A, et al. Maternal Lyme disease and congenital malformation: a cord blood serosurvey in endemic and control arcas. Paediatr Perinat Epidemiol. 1995;9:320–30.

Leonard H. Sigal, MD

A Vaccine Recipient Who Develops Arthralgia and Fatigue

A 54-year-old man, who received the Lyme vaccine in May, presents to his family physician in July with the chief symptom of arthralgias and fatigue. He lives in an area endemic for Lyme disease and spends a great deal of time outdoors, but he denies a history of a tick bite, erythema migrans, fever, stiff neck, or facial palsy. He also denies nasal congestion, sore throat, or abdominal symptoms. His past medical history is significant for mild hypertension.

On physical examination, he is afebrile. His blood pressure is 150/86 mm Hg and his pulse rate is 80 beats/min. His skin is without rash. His HEENT examinations is unremarkable. His lungs are clear, his heart rate is regular, and heart rhythm is without rubs or murmurs. His abdominal examination is benign. His musculoskeletal examination is notable for tenderness of the medial aspect of both knees and crepitance during range of motion. His neurologic examination yields nonfocal findings.

Laboratory studies performed at the time of presentation include a leukocyte count of 5900/mm^3 with a normal differential. His hemoglobin was 13.9 and hematocrit was 39.3%. He had normal electrolytes, liver function studies, and cholesterol level. Uric acid was 6.3 mg/dL. Monospot test, rheumatoid factor, antistreptolysin titer, and antinuclear antibody titers are negative. His sedimentation rate is 3 mm/h. Lyme enzyme-linked immunosorbent assay (ELISA) results obtained at a commercial laboratory are interpreted as positive.

■ QUESTION

Is this patient's presentation compatible with Lyme disease?

■ COMMENT

This patient presents with nonspecific symptoms, including arthralgias and fatigue. Although he lives in an area endemic for Lyme disease, these findings by themselves do not point to the diagnosis of Lyme disease.

The risks of a false-positive serologic test result in this patient will be significant because the prevalence of Lyme disease in such individuals is low. More importantly, this patient has already received a Lyme disease vaccine. Because of this, he will have antibodies against the 31-kd OspA *Borrelia burgdorferi* protein. These antibodies will be detected by the Lyme ELISA and will generate a positive test result.

In the absence of specific clinical features suggesting a diagnosis of Lyme disease, the best course of action may be not to do serologic testing for Lyme disease at all. If such testing is to be done in a person who has received the Lyme disease vaccine, it will need to be sent to a laboratory where Western blot analysis can be done that omits the 31-kd response.

■ CONCLUSION

In Lyme disease recipients, Western blot analysis is indicated to distinguish disease from seroconversion caused by vaccination.

Wormser GP. A vaccine against Lyme disease [editorial]? Ann Intern Med. 1995; 123:627–9.
Wormser GP. Lyme disease vaccine. Infection. 1996;24:203–7.

Robert T. Schoen, MD

Appendix

■　■　■

FDA Public Health Advisory: Assays for Antibodies to *Borrelia burgdorferi*; Limitations, Use, and Interpretation for Supporting a Clinical Diagnosis of Lyme Disease

Purpose

FDA is advising you about the potential for misdiagnosis of Lyme disease. The results of commonly marketed assays for detecting antibody to *Borrelia burgdorferi* (anti-*Bb*), the organism that causes Lyme disease, may be easily misinterpreted. To reduce this risk of misdiagnosis, we are providing guidance on the use and interpretation of these tests. It is important that clinicians understand the limitations of these tests. A positive result does not necessarily indicate current infection with *B. burgdorferi*, and patients with active Lyme disease may have a negative test result (1–5).

Assays for anti-*Bb* should be used only to support a clinical diagnosis of Lyme disease. Physicians are advised to base diagnosis on history (including symptoms and exposure to the tick vector), physical findings, and laboratory data other than anti-*Bb* results. The most definitive diagnostic procedure, biopsy and isolation in culture, frequently yields organism when collection and culture procedures are optimal but often is not practical. Assays for anti-*Bb* can provide evidence of previous or current infection; however, to improve reliability, **results should be interpreted only in the context of a two-step testing algorithm (described below) and should not, by themselves, be used to establish a diagnosis of Lyme disease or to exclude *Bb* infection.** The two-step algorithm, as opposed to using a single test, increases the specificity of laboratory testing.

Although package inserts for some commercial assays describe their intended use "to aid in the diagnosis of Lyme disease," this statement does not fully reflect current knowledge about *Bb* infections, and many such assays yield potentially misleading results. FDA is applying the following recommendations as it works with manufacturers to change package inserts and as it evaluates new assays for anti-*Bb*.

Recommendations for Two-Step Testing and Interpretation of Results

The FDA Microbiology Advisory Panel has advised that package inserts of anti-*Bb* assays should promote the two-step testing algorithm recommended by the Second National Conference on Serologic Diagnosis of Lyme Disease (1,2), which included representatives from the Centers for Disease Control and Prevention (CDC), the Association of State and Territorial Public Health Laboratory Directors, manufacturers of assays, academic researchers, and FDA.

- The first step is to perform an assay that detects either total or class-specific antibodies (IgM or IgG) by using enzyme-linked immunosorbent technology ("ELISA" or "EIA") or indirect immunofluoresence microscopy ("IFA"). IgM levels usually peak 3 to 6 weeks after infection. IgG antibodies begin to be detectable several weeks after infection. The IgG response may continue to develop over the course of several months and generally persists for years.
  - A negative result indicates that there was not serologic evidence of infection with *Bb* at the time the specimen was collected. A negative result should not be the basis for excluding *Bb* as the cause of illness, especially if blood was collected within 2 weeks of when symptoms began. If Lyme disease is strongly suspected, a second specimen should be collected 2 to 4 weeks after the first specimen and then tested.
  - A positive or equivocal result is presumptive evidence of the presence of anti-*Bb*, should always be followed by second-step testing, and should not be reported until second-step testing is complete.
- The second step employs an assay that is more specific than that used for the first step. To date, Western-blot (immunoblot) assays have been used for second-step testing. This second test is more specific than ELISA or IFA because Western blot determines if serum contains antibodies (IgG or IgM) that react with appropriate *Bb* antigens separated by electrophoresis.
  - A negative result indicates that no reliable serologic evidence of *Bb* infection was present at the time the specimen was collected. A negative result should not be the sole basis for ex-

cluding *Bb* as the cause of illness. If Lyme disease is strongly suspected, a second specimen collected 2 to 4 weeks after the first specimen should be tested.

- A positive result provides serologic evidence of past or current infection with *Bb*. Because the presence of even specific antibodies to *Bb* does not always indicate current infection, a positive result can support, but not establish, a clinical diagnosis of Lyme disease.

While this algorithm is a consensus approach for detecting serologic evidence of infection with *Bb*, the sensitivity and specificity of both steps are less than optimal. Physicians may be familiar with other two-step testing algorithms, such as that for antibodies to human immunodeficiency virus, in which a highly sensitive first-step assay is sometimes referred to as a "screening" test and a highly specific second-step assay as "confirmatory." Because assays for anti-*Bb* should be used only for supporting a clinical diagnosis of Lyme disease and not for "screening" asymptomatic individuals, "initial" is preferred for describing the first step. Second-step Western-blot assays are "supplemental" rather than "confirmatory" because of suboptimal specificity, particularly for detecting IgM anti-*Bb*. Thus, a positive IgM anti-*Bb* result alone is not recommended for supporting a diagnosis of Lyme disease in persons with illness of greater than 1 month duration (1,2).

Background Information

Several important factors contribute to the limitations of using ELISA, IFA, or Western-blot tests for supporting Lyme disease diagnosis. The stage of disease in which the specimen was taken is critical. First, many patients with active or recent infections do not have detectable anti-*Bb* in a single specimen. This happens because such antibodies often develop subsequent to manifestations of early infection (the majority of patients' sera are negative for IgM anti-*Bb* at presentation, whereas most will have detectable IgM and/or IgG anti-*Bb* if sera are collected and tested at both presentation and 2 to 4 weeks later) or because detectable anti-*Bb* may diminish or never develop in patients treated with antibacterial drugs. Secondly, it is not possible to make a definite temporal association between detectable anti-*Bb* and an illness because these antibodies do not indicate when infection with *Bb* occurred or if there is active Lyme disease. Serologic assays can detect anti-*Bb* for many years after infection. Thus, a positive result can be true evidence of previous infection with *Bb*, unrelated to current illness. Finally, assays for anti-*Bb* frequently yield false-positive results because of cross-reactive antibodies associated with autoimmune diseases or from infection with other spirochetes, rickettsia, ehrlichia, or other bacteria such as *Helicobacter pylori* (5–7).

Reporting Adverse Events to FDA

Physicians are encouraged to report adverse events related to medical devices, including clinical laboratory assays, to MedWatch, the voluntary program for reporting to FDA. Pertinent adverse events could include anti-*Bb* results that led to inappropriate management or a problem with quality control of an assay. Submit these reports by telephone to 1-800-FDA-1088, by fax to 1-800-FDA-0178, or by mail to MedWatch, Food and Drug Administration, HF-2, 5600 Fishers Lane, Rockville, MD 20857.

Getting More Information

If you have any questions regarding this Advisory, please contact John Ticehurst, MD, or Roxanne Shively, CDRH, Office of Device Evaluation, HFZ-440, 2098 Gaither Road, Rockville, MD 20850, or FAX 301-594-5941. Please include your phone number with any correspondence.

> Sincerely yours,
> D. Bruce Burlington, M.D.
> Director
> Center for Devices and
>   Radiological Health

REFERENCES

1. Centers for Disease Control and Prevention. Recommendations for test performance and interpretation from the second national conference on serologic diagnosis of Lyme disease. MMWR. 1995;44:590-1.
2. Association of State and Territorial Public Health Laboratory Directors and the Centers for Disease Control and Prevention. Recommendations. In: Proceedings of the Second National Conference on Serologic Diagnosis of Lyme Disease (Dearborn, Michigan). Washington, DC: Association of State and Territorial Public Health Laboratory Directors 1995;1-5.
3. **Craven RB, Quan TJ, Bailey RE, et al.** Improved seriodiagnostic testing for Lyme disease: results of a multicenter serologic evaluation. Emerg Infect Dis. 1996;2:136-40.
4. **Bakken LL, Callister SM, Wand PJ, Schell RF.** Interlaboratory comparison of test results for detection of Lyme disease by 516 participants in the Wisconsin State Laboratory of Hygiene/College of American Pathologists proficiency testing program. J Clin Microbiol. 1997;35:537-43.
5. **Johnson RC, Johnson BJB.** Lyme disease: serodiagnosis of *Borrelia burgdorferi sensu lato* infection. In Rose NR, Macario EC, Fahey JL, et al, eds. Manual of Clinical Laboratory Immunology. 5th ed. Washington, DC: American Society for Microbiology, 1997:526-33.

6. **Magnarelli LA, Miller JN, Anderson JF, Riviere GR.** Cross-reactivity of nonspecific treponemal antibody in serologic tests for Lyme disease. J Clin Microbiol. 1990;28:1276-9.

7. **Schwan TG, Burgdorfer W, Rosa PA.** Borrelia. In: Murray PR, Baron EJ, Pfaller MA, et al, eds. Manual of Clinical Microbiology. 6th ed. Washington DC: American Society for Microbiology, 1995:626-35.

Index

Color Plates

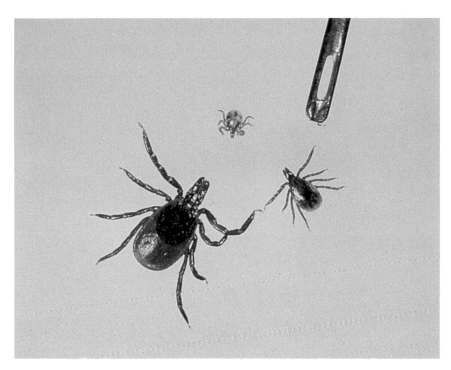

Plate 1 The three life forms (larva, nymph, adult) of unfed *Ixodes scapularis,* the black-legged (deer) tick. Their sizes are shown relative to the eye of a sewing needle. Nymphs, which feed during late spring and early summer, are responsible for most cases of Lyme disease. (Courtesy of Russell C. Johnson, PhD, University of Minnesota.) See discussion of Figure 1.3 in Chapter 1 text (Plate 1 reproduced in black and white) for further information.

Continued

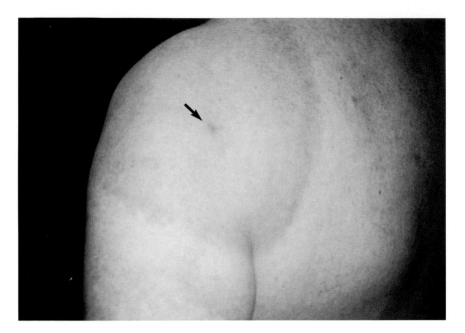

Plate 2 Erythema migrans rash with central clearing on the shoulder of a patient. Note central hyperpigmentation at site of tick bite (punctum) (*arrow*). *Borrelia burgdorferi* was isolated from a biopsy culture performed at the periphery of the lesion. (Reprinted with permission from Nadelman RB, Wormser GP. Erythema migrans and early Lyme disease. Am J Med. 1995;98(suppl 4A): 15S-24S.) See discussion of Figure 3.1 in Chapter 3 text (Plate 2 reproduced in black and white) for further information.

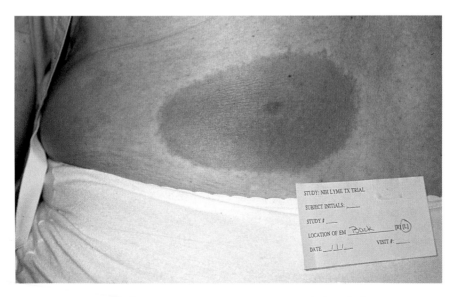

Plate 3 Erythema migrans rash without central clearing. *Borrelia burgdorferi* was isolated from a biopsy culture performed at the periphery of the lesion. See discussion of Figure 3.2 in Chapter 3 text (Plate 3 reproduced in black and white) for further information.

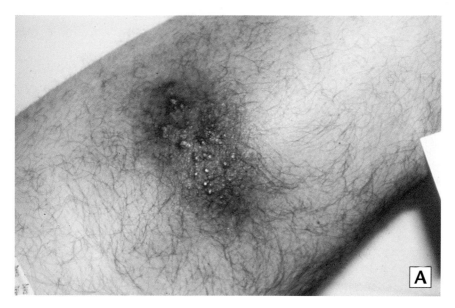

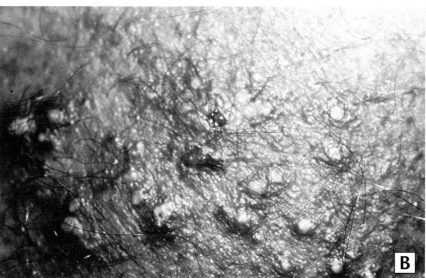

Plate 4 *A,* Vesicular erythema migrans (EM) lesion. *B,* Close-up of same vesicular EM lesion. *Borrelia burgdorferi* was isolated from culture from vesicular fluid. (Reprinted with permission from Nadelman RB, Wormser GP. Erythema migrans and early Lyme disease. Am J Med. 1995; 98(suppl 4A): 15S-24S.) See discussion of Figure 3.3 in Chapter 3 text (Plate 4 reproduced in black and white) for further information.

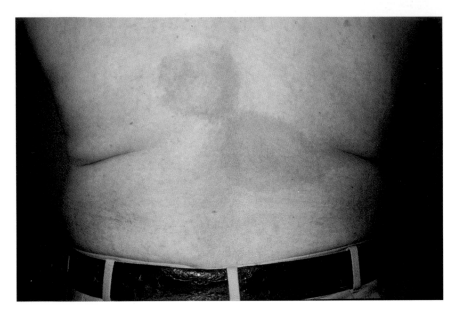

Plate 5 Multiple erythema migrans lesions on the back of a patient whose primary lesion is depicted in Plate 2. Note the absence of a central papule or postinflammatory skin change. (Reprinted with permission from Nadelman RB, Wormser GP. Erythema migrans and early Lyme disease. Am J Med. 1995;98(suppl 4A): 15S-24S.) See discussion of Figure 3.4 in Chapter 3 text (Plate 5 reproduced in black and white) for further information.

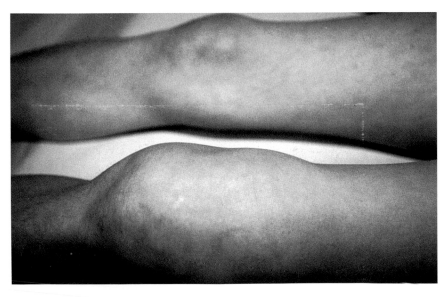

Plate 6 Unilateral knee effusion in Lyme arthritis. See discussion of Figure 6.1 in Chapter 6 text (Plate 6 reproduced in black and white) for further information.